Songs of Destiny

BY

Lydia Li Olson

Songs of Destiny

American Success Publishing
San Francisco, CA
Phone: +1 (510)366-5166
Email: asp665166@gmail.com

ISBN: 979-8-9866845-9-8
Printed in the United States of America

Contents

Editor's Note

This book is the autobiography of a Chinese woman. The work tells a story spanning two centuries, three marriages, three cancers, and the experience of being deeply influenced and impacted by the cultures of China and the United States, which can give people inspiration, reflection and reference.

The history is of the author's Manchu family and the story of her own growth in Beijing, sometimes in conflict the author's own personality. Especially during the Cultural Revolution, true thoughts and deeds were incompatible with the atmosphere of the time. The author describes in detail how to work in the artillery farm, how to adapt herself to the harsh environment around her as much as possible in the third-line ravines of Guizhou, and the details of meeting close friends and facing tortuous work transfers. It is a true and vivid reflection of the Chinese society at that time.

The second half is even more undulating, from the interpreter at foreign embassies in Beijing, the happy family, to the embarrassing scene of family breakdown and lone struggle, the pain of broken marriage, and the intersecting experience of struggles in the United States all are lamentable. The writing is concise and vivid. During the Cultural Revolution, she left in anger at the criticism and the beating of her teacher, rode a bicycle to the hospital alone before giving birth, suffered from cancer chemotherapy twice and lost her hair, and jokingly called herself a nun. The stubborn character of a Manchu woman who dares to love and dares to take actions, and not accept defeat, is very apparent.

Studying in the United States, it was said she was a woman who betrayed the motherland, but she has been attached to the motherland all her life, loving and inheriting Chinese culture like a consistent red thread throughout the loom of her life. At Lake Houhai, Beijing, she learned Tai Chi, understood the essence of Chinese culture. Deep in the mountains and valleys, she used Tai Chi to drive away depression and loneliness. In California she taught Tai Chi, Tai Chi sword, Chinese lessons giving students a chance to understand Chinese culture, especially the ceremony she designed for the death of her father-in-law, She asked her American husband, the U.S Army military band trumpeter, to play her father's favorite music when he was cremated, and then, she and her husband performed 24 movement Tai Chi together which was very touching. This book is the first book published by the author, and the manuscript was praised as soon as it came out.

Zhang Zhong-Qing

Publisher and Chief Editor, Mandarin Version American Success Publishing

"Every life is a journey of discovery, learning, struggle, awakening, joy, sorrow, love, loss, and suffering. Here, Lydia Li Olson recounts all those things in the dual life she led, half in China and the other half in the United States. Her cross-cultural journey proves beyond any doubt, that those experiences are common to every culture and every soul. They are our shared humanity as we navigate the mystery of what it means to be fully alive, embracing every life circumstance with courage and hope. Reading Lydia's story will certainly shed much light on your own. A marvelous and deeply emotional memoir!"

- John Schettler, English Version Editor, The Writing Shop Press

Overture

Farewell to Arthur Dieli, my Father-in-law

My third husband Daniel's father was a full-blooded Italian, born in Connecticut, USA, named Arthur Dieli. He studied law, computers, and was proficient in several languages. He retired as a computer professor from a university in California. I had known him for 11 years and admired him from the bottom of my heart. He was knowledgeable and well-learned. When he took Daniel and I on a tour to Sicily as a honeymoon, we met the relatives of the Dieli family. He introduced me to the local history, culture, architecture, religion, and food. Arthur died in Sacramento, California's Capital, on March 19, 2019, at the age of 92. As he lay dying, he endured with astonishing perseverance until Daniel and I rushed back to him from Italy on March 18 and then he passed away peacefully after we arrived 8 hours. The husband of Daniel's sister, Jorge, picked us from San Francisco airport at 2 am in the morning told us that he couldn't believe our father hang on there for over two days waiting for Daniel and I arrive. Jorge said any other old man would have stopped breathing on Sunday when he passed out. I thank the Higher Power arranged the time for us to bid bye to each other.

I've always been afraid of the dead. Even when my own

father and mother died, I didn't dare to touch their bodies. But for some reason, I didn't have any feeling of fear for my father in-law's critically ill and deceased body. I was able to hold his hand and kiss his forehead. I said to his ear that we came back to visit him from Italy,

The wife of one of Daniel's cousins, Cathy, said to me, "You know what? Arthur told me quite a few times when he was alive that he liked you very much and valued you very much. He said you changed his son's life." I am very glad that Cathy passed the words to me. Otherwise, I didn't know why my father-in-law liked us to visit him so much and always had big smiles when he saw me. Before we arrived at his house in Sacramento, he had the bed made already. Clean towers hanged in the bathroom. He cooked breakfast for us before we got up. He cooked Italian pasta for us for dinner or lunch. He also used his fancy looking Italian machine to make cappuccino for us. I also learned from him to put fruits in yogurt which tasted great. He also picked up sweet figs, cherries, oranges and lemon from his yard for me. In 2013, at the age of 86 Arthur led his fifth daughter Sara's whole family to San Mateo to see me perform the Peking opera Farewell My Concubine despite he had a sharp pain on his leg. I was very moved.

His will was to die without any funeral or memorial service. All his daughters obeyed. When his body was taken away from the house, nobody said a word or cried. His daughters and son and his grandchildren all stand inside the two sides of garage. I asked aloud, "That's it? We won't see him again. No ceremony?" Sister Paula said, "Yes, That's it. That is what Dad wanted. We have to follow his instructions." I burst into tears and knelled down in front of the funeral car. I kowtowed to him three times. And then the car went away. When we came back to the house I found Arthurs' care-giver for the last two weeks, a black young man (sorry I forgot his name) stood at the backyard sobbing. He covered his face with his hands and his body was shaking. I walked to him and so did other siters. He was very sad and told us, "I love him and never expect him to only stay with me for two weeks. I have never met any my patients so gentle and kind. Every day he told me stories of his life and every one of you. I had such a good time coming here. I already miss him "

Daniel was very sad but didn't say a word. On the day of father's cremation at the balcony of a friend's house in the San Francisco Bay Area, facing the Pacific Ocean of San Francisco Bay, I created a farewell ceremony for Arthur. Daniel played three of his father's favorite pieces of music on the trumpet: the first was Aranjuez by the Spanish composer Joaquin Rodrigo. This piece is one of the most famous classical guitar pieces in the world. The second was Back to Sorrento by Italian composer, Ernesto De Curtis. The third was the Hungarian composer Joseph Kosma's Autumn Leaves based on the French poet Jacques Prevert, whose melodies are world-famous. All show a deep sense of homesickness and longing. Daniel's expression when he played the trumpet was solemn and full of passion.. The sounds he blew out were magnificent and sad. The sound went straight to the sky. I believed that day when Arthur's soul went to heaven, he must have heard that solo trumpet from his only son (Danie had three older siters and three younger sisters. We all get together at Christmas or Thanksgiving-what a nice family!)

I burst into tears as I listened to the three pieces that Daniel played for his father. If Arthur was still alive, I could see he would have tears in his eyes. I could also see his smiling and satisfied facial expression, very proud of his son. After Daniel finished playing the trumpet, I sang with deep emotion Ave Maria which I studied in Italy from Victoria Lyamina, a mezzo soprano from Moscow. In the end, we both played 24-style Tai Chi three times. I remembered Arthur was very happy to watch me and Daniel perform Tai Chi and Tai Chi sword together. I am very happy to arrange this farewell ceremony to our father in a special way to comfort the spirit of him in heaven and give us a chance to pay tribute to his glorious life and also leaves no regret in my heart.

The sound of Daniel's trumpet was rippling over the sky of the San Francisco Bay Area. I could see the vast Pacific Ocean. Its swelling blue waves reached all the way to China on the other side of the Pacific Ocean. It also connects me to my first kiss, my first love, my first husband Wang Bing-sheng. They are all there, in Beijing, the capital of China.

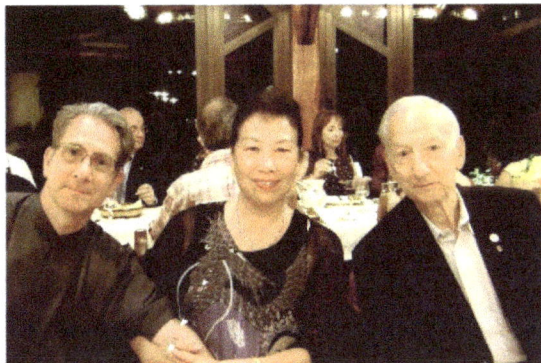

Chapter 1

My First Love My Husband My Big Tree

After working on the farm over a year, Wang Bingsheng was selected to study at Beijing Foreign Language Institute. Then he was assigned to work at the Kuwaiti Embassy stationed in Beijing.

My Prince Charming, Wang Bingsheng, was born in a beautiful city called Qingdao, in Shan dong Province, where the Chinese Ballet School went in search of male students. He is 6 feet tall, with big eyes, a high bridge nose, well-shaped mouth, neither fat or skinny. He is very stylish in any clothes, and one can sense his well-versed knowledge and impartial views in his conversation. We two worked in the same company after I was transferred back to Beijing from Guizhou. He was so clever that he remembers everything even if he only read something one time. Like my mother-in-law, he has a kind heart, and would rather suffer losses himself to let others get by. No matter where he goes, he has an excellent reputation.

There is a certain karma relationship between people, and there is fate between people arranged by destiny. Wang Bing sheng and I were admitted to The Preparatory Course of the Beijing Foreign Trade Institute (equivalent to high school) at the same year. There were 6 classes of English, and later we were divided into classes according to the result of study scores. We two were both assigned to No. 3 class composed of higher scoring students. There were student representatives for each class. Bing sheng was the representative of the geometry class and I was the representative of Chinese Language and Physical Education class. There was no deep friendship between the two of us, but no differences between us either. We were not childhood sweethearts, but we had mutual respect because he was a very smart student who didn't need to study hard to obtain good grades.

I stood out from the crowd in every subject. After three years of study in school, we were both accepted to the same university but in different departments located in two different places (now known as University ofInternational Business and Economics). Mine was inside the city near my home while his was in the west suburbs of Beijing. We didn't have much communication after entering the university, but our teachers were in competition behind the scene because the two classes were all composed by the higher score students. However, a few years later, fate brought us together and formed a happy family that everyone envied. Isn't this what Chinese colloquialism said: "It takes hundred years to ride the same boat, thousand years to sleep on the same pillow?"

When I returned to Beijing from Guizhou to visit my family, I rode my bike to Haidian District to deliver a train ticket to an old mother of the military representative who worked in my factory because the military representative entrusted me to bring his old mother back to Guizhou. On the way back, a group of plainly dressed students called my name. When I looked back, I saw that my old classmates from the preparatory course and the university had just returned from a labor field, a total of eight of them! After I left Beijing to go to the farm, I never heard anything from them, let alone met them. Now I suddenly met them on the road in Haidian District. As if we were family members who had not seen each other for many years, they warmly invited me to Beijing Foreign Language University where they were assigned to re-study English. I learned that after graduation, they were sent to Tangshan Farm to be re-educated through farm labor. Now they were chosen to further their English studies and then assigned to be interpreters.

To make the long story short, it seemed that most of my

classmates were in the process of dating or married with children. Only Wang Bing-sheng and I were single. His English teacher, Zhang Bing-zi, and my English teacher, Zhang Yin-yu, secretly competed to see who's students were taught better. I heard that before the Cultural Revolution, the school selected several students from our two classes to take the examination for study abroad. The first place in the oral test was Wang Bing sheng of Zhang Bing-zi's class, and the first place in the written test was Chen Zhen-yu of my teacher Zhang Yinyu's class. It was a draw. However the Cultural Revolution started after that. Their opportunities to study abroad were also blown.

Is man's life predestined? In schools, on farms, or in factories there were several male college graduates with good reputations. They were from my school Beijing Foreign Trade Institute or Beijing University, or Qinghua University, or Ha Er Bin Military Industry University, and so on. Quite a few young men directly or indirectly wanted to have a date with me. Maybe, my physiological level and age were not on the same line, or my desire for men was delayed, or maybe I didn't have an eye for any of them. I was 26 years old and I was still single. The Prince Charming in my heart did not appear for a long time. Everyone around me was anxious and worried that I might not be able to marry. But I never lost faith - my Prince Charming would come one day.

Who would have thought that on the main road in Beijing's Haidian District, from nowhere he appeared! Since we graduated, we had no contact and didn't know each other's situation. After this coincidence and a hint from a schoolmate, Wang Bing-sheng and I began to correspond as boy and girl friends. Flipping through the photo albums, several pictures of my teenage years, whether it was the whole class together or the class representatives together, he always stood next to me (this was discovered by mt friends .). Isn't that fate? It seems a little strange that we were suddenly in love, but it was smooth sailing. The mutual understanding and mutual respect and admiration for each other since we were 15 years old in the same class planted the seeds and laid the foundation. I believe Karma.

The next year, I returned to Beijing on my annual leave to meet him "officially." He had been assigned the ChiefInterpreter at the Kuwaiti Embassy in China. His working unit was called Beijing Diplomatic Service Bureau under the Ministry of Foreign Affairs. The official title of interpreters who worked in the foreign embassies were all called "Chinese Secretary."

The first time he came to my house from work, I wasn't home. Later, as soon as I entered the door, I saw my second elder sister was overjoyed and excitedly said to me, "Just now Wang Bingsheng came to visit. I haven't seen him since you two graduated from the Preparatory Course of Beijing Foreign Trade Institute, I didn't expect him to grow so tall, completely different from when he was a young man in high school. I remembered when you two were in The Preparatory Course class, I went to see you. A young man with fair skin, wearing a Chinese traditional coat, shouted with a voice like a clown, 'Li Chongjun (my born name), someone outside is looking for you!' I was so impressed with his good looks and humorous manner. Now he still looks much the same, only he is taller, more handsome and personable. I was overjoyed and then my sister said: 'I'm glad you two are dating now."

For several years, my second elder sister had been looking for a boyfriend for me, but I seemed to be indifferent. Not having a boyfriend had also become a burden in my mother's heart. Several times my mother angrily "reprimanded" me, "Do you know how old you are? You know nothing but to play all day long. Why don't you give a thought about your personal matters? When are you going to stop playing?" I replied naughtily, "Yes, I love to play. I'll still keep playing even when I'm eighty." Now my prince Charm came to my life. I was very happy to see that both my mother and my isster like Wang Bingsheng so much.

Our first date was at my favorite, the Summer Palace. Seeing him had grown from a much shorter young man to a handsome gentleman who was much taller than me, my heart was filled with joy, which I had never had before. My second elder sister, her husband, their daughter Jingjing, and my best friend from great school, all came to join us on that day. Bingsheng didn't mind at all. Getting along with everyone in a humble way, he was generous, polite and well-behaved. I was filled with good feelings and had great respect for him. At the Summer Palace, we took unforgettable photos.

He is a truly manly husband, extremely intelligent, humorous and witty, super insightful, personable, handsome, sincere, true in love, persistent in love. Since I grew up, he was my first love and the first kiss was so sweet that I would never forget!

Nixon's visit to China in 1972 began a new chapter in the history of China and the United States. Premier Zhou asked,

"Where are all the interpreters we trained?" The chief of the Human Resource Department of the Diplomatic Service Bureau under the Ministry of Foreign Affairs, where Bingsheng worked, knew about our relationship, met me, and conducted an English examination of my English level. They are very satisfied with my English. The personnel department immediately decided to transfer me to the Beijing Diplomatic Service Bureau from the factory where I was working in the deep mountain in Keli, Guizhou. Before I returned to the factory, the transfer order was already arrived for me to go back to Beijing to report to the Human Resource office of the Ministry of Foreign Affairs.

As for the setbacks I painfully experienced in the subsequent transfer work, it will be described later in details. In the blink of an eye, two years had passed. During those years, Bingsheng and I wrote letters in English once a week, pouring out each other's thoughts and our views oflife. When I returned to Beijing to visit my family, Wang Bingsheng relayed his family's wish: It is time to get married. My vanity made me feel that it was disgraceful to transfer back to Beijing by relying on a wife's identity. I should have been transferred back to Beijing because of the needs of foreign affairs work, so I was a little hesitant to get married. The eldest sister of Bingsheng persuaded me, "If you two are married, that is a better reason to be transferred back to Beijing." She was four years older than me, a graduate from the Physics Department of Beijing University and worked as a chief engineer at a Beijing electronic factory. She liked me and I always respected her. Even after I separated from Bingsheng for various reasons, I had always maintained contact and friendly relationships with her. I discussed with my mother and second elder sister about the marriage. They liked Bingsheng and had no objections, I agreed.

The leader of the Diplomatic Service Bureau found us a room where female staff lived who left for Chinese New Year vacation. My second elder sister and my younger sister were busy preparing bedding and basic daily necessities. The wedding was scheduled at Bingsheng parents' house, and no one except members of the two families were present. We got married right before China's New Year.

How to bring everything from my home to the borrowed bridal chamber? It was my junior high school classmate, Hou Yu-Ian, who rode a tricycle to take my luggage to Beijing Railway when I first left home for Shandong Artillery Farm to be re educated through farm labor (You will read that story later). The second interesting thing in our marriage was that the location of the bridal chamber was recognized by my second elder sister. That was the building where I went to kindergarten when I was four or five years old! She told me it was the kindergarten she had found for me, which was run by the United States General Relief Administration after the Second World War in Beijing. It was a kindergarten for Chinese children to eat lunch and attend classes at no cost. Every day she sent me in the morning and picked me up in the afternoon.

I still remembered a scene: the first time when I went to the kindergarten, which was a two-storied building I was not used to walking on stairs and I rolled down. When I mentioned it, my second elder sister said, "For some reason you always fell down when you were a child. You were also often easily knocked down by other people. When you fell, you fainted and frightened me several times." We both laughed. She said, "I also remembered there was a teacher, Ms. Hu, in the kindergarten, who especially liked you because you learned to sing and dance quickly."

When I grew up, I heard people say that life was a circle. I didn't expect that the place where I went to kindergarten at the age of four or five would become my bridal chamber! Later, I went to work in the Commercial Office of the US Embassy in China, came to California in 1987 to study, and now I have an American husband and we live in the most beautiful place in California. I certainly had good Karma in the United States!

After less than twenty days of staying in my bridal chamber where we had an unforgettable time, the leader of the Human Resource office informed us that the ladies of the house would return soon, and he had found another place for us to spend our honeymoon. My royal "tricycle driver" Hou Yulan came to help again. She said, "What's going on? How come you have to move before the honeymoon is over?" I said that Bingsheng and I were already grateful to have a place to get married. Fortunately, we didn't have much except for the bedding and some personal belongings. When we arrived at my second bridal chamber, we all laughed. We were looking at a greenhouse of the former Japanese Embassy in Suzhou Lane near Beijing Railway Station. There were large glass panels on three sides, but fortunately the green house was located in a large courtyard in the backyard. There were no neighbors next to it. The two of us continued our honeymoon. We didn't care it was once a greenhouse. Unforgettable and sweet memories remains forever.

I had to go back to Guizhou in early March. Later, my annual leave became the only precious time we could see each other. I remembered that every time I entered the railroad station on the train from Guizhou to Beijing, I could see that handsome figure standing at the first platform. It was him, my husband, whom I missed day and night! I always opened the window of the train eagerly looking for that familiar face. After he saw me from the window of the train, he ran with the train, reached in from outside the window and took my hand. The joy of our love cannot be described in words. Whenever

I left Beijing and had to return to Guizhou, he bought packages of snacks that I grew up with. When I thought that I would soon have to leave him, I couldn't stop crying. He always comforted me and said, " To be sad is useless, and time will pass quickly. Dawn is ahead.." One year after we got married, Bing-sheng accompanied me back to Kaili, Guizhou where I worked or suffered for 7-8 years. Although he was a year younger than me, he always took care of me like a big brother. The factory gave us a temporary family dormitory. He didn't go anywhere every day, using limited supplies to make breakfast, lunch and dinner. Although the conditions were very difficult, he always laughed and made humorous jokes from time to time, temporarily ending the bitterness of my single life. Before I left work for our temporary home, I felt very happy because I didn't have to go back to the singles dormitory, but to the family area, back to the warm little family, back to his side. He is like a bright moon, which makes me feel peaceful; he was like a sunny sun, which makes me feel warm. In fact, he is a big tree around me, so that I always have a sense of security and dependence. It seems life is like a big mountain on my shoulder, but I am not afraid, because he carries it for me.

The deep friendship and indescribable conjugal love between us is touching. It's never going away. These are my wonderful memories.

He is indeed a towering tree in my heart, a manly husband with dignity! I lost him! For ten years, the bitter regret lingered in my heart. Pain and helplessness pushed me into an abyss. In the next life, I will choose him as my husband again because he is not only a man who stands tall in the world, but also a good husband who loved his wife, took care of his wife, and loves his children and teaches them as a good father. In my next life I am also willing to be a big tree, grow firm and tall in the world and breathe freely. I would grow into a tall tree that will make my loved ones and my children and grandchildren take shelter from the wind and the rain, live peacefully, and never separate.

Some people questioned me, "What is the use of writing this? After all, you two are separated now!" Over the years, through studying, listening to lectures by masters, and observing the relationship between the people around me, I feel that the three-dimensional world we live in is too small, too bland, too rigid, and too limited. The universe is unimaginable to us and the relationships between people are complex. They are subject to many constraints, unattainable, unsettled by human will, and unpredictable. There is a heavy word a mysterious world. There is a name is called Fate. The radio waves that flow among people are an energy. This energy will bring us eternal power. It inspires me to always move forward. Writing down all these happenings in detail, remembering the sweet time, looking back on the years of sharing happiness and hardship with Bingsheng filled my heart with gratitude. The pain has passed, leaving behind an inexhaustible amount of energy.

Sometimes it seems I was still in dream: How come a spoiled Manchu girl became a lucky woman who had a happy family everyone admired? How come this happy family disappeared after 16 years? Mystery, mystery and mystery.

Wang Bingsheng (Ice) my first husband

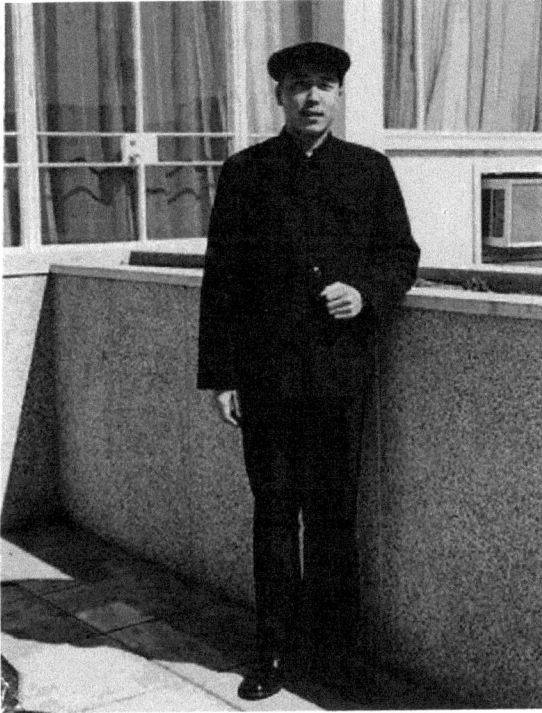

Chapter 2

I am from A Manchu Family

I've never seen my grandpa or grandma. I heard that my grandfather's name was Li Yuechuan, who served in the Imperial Palace (Gu Gong) known as the Forbidden City. Now it is called The Palace Museum. He was the head of Luan Yi Wei in the Imperial Palace equivalent of a protocol department. He was in charge of what sedan would be used for the activities of the Emperor's family, such as birthdays, weddings, office visits, private activities; how many people would carry the sedan, what kind of music would be played, and what kinds of flags would be held, etc. He worked for Chinese rulers, such as Empress Dowager Cixi, Emperor Guang Xu, the last emperor Puyi. In modern terms, my grandfather's job was called "Director of the Royal Protocol Department of the Imperial Palace ." He was given the allowance equivalent to a third-rank official.

The Li family was a branch of the Yellow Banner also known as Ai Xin Jue Luo. My ancestors had served the emperors' family for generations. My younger sister has in her hand a photograph of my grandfather at the age of 56, tall, dressed in a robe, with a serious face, typical of a Manchu old man. From several of our descendants, one can see we inherited his physiognomy, such as the shape of his mouth, teeth and eyes. When a few of us stand together, we are living examples of the descendants of the Li family.

Grandpa's address is written in ink at the back side of this photo. Address: No. 7, Yang Jiao Deng Hutong, Beiping (the old name of Peking or Beijing) which is near to the Forbidden City when he was 56 years old. Three years after taking the photo, Grandpa died at the age of 59. My father also died at the age of 59 when I was 17 years old.

My father was the eldest in Li's family. He had two younger sisters, my second and third aunts who loved me very much. Grandma died when my father was only fourteen years old. His two sisters were only 5 and 3 years old. Grandpa never married a second wife because he was afraid that his two daughters might have a hard time with a stepmother. When my second aunt told me about these stories of the Li family, I was full of respect for my grandfather whom I had only seen in a photo.

The last Emperor Puyi stepped down in 1911 and was forced to move out of the Imperial Palace in 1924. The Eight Banners' Manchu people who did not have any worries about eating and clothes before now lost their allowances. They had no job skills, so they had to go to the pawnshop to pawn what they could to make a living.

Mom was 19 when she married Dad. I remembered when I was in junior high school, my neighbor Mrs. Bai came to my house to chat with Mom. I heard Mom said, "When I got married, the people who came out to see my palanquin occupied the two sides of the streets." I asked why and my mother proudly said, "Yes, the people who carried the palanquin for me were all from the Imperial Palace carrying palanquins for the emperor's family. Your grandfather was the head of Luan Yi Wei (The section where all the sedans and banners were kept for the emperor's family)." Mrs. Bai said admirably, "Of course, the head ofLuan Yi Wei welcomes his daughter-in-law to Li's family, who else would have such an honor to sit inside the palanquin?" Mrs. Bai also said to me, "Third girl, you are not blessed to enjoy such a day when you marry. You are no longer a Gege (Gege is the pronunciation of princess referring to the girls of a Manchu family before she is married)."

I can imagine my mother's grandeur at that time: she was 5'4, a standard height with double eyelids and a pair of beautiful eyes and her mouth was neither big or small with perfect shape. Her complexion was fair, a quasi-beauty. How nice it would have been to have a camera at that time. Unfortunately, my mother's stylish image did not even leave a photo. Now when I see people acting or taking pictures of people wearing Manchu costumes, I will put wings of imagination on the scene when my mother got married. It was a picture without a photo. It was a movie without a videotape. Mom told me that when she got married, the 8 rooms of Li's family were filled with carved red lacquer furniture and a variety of porcelain and antiques. I asked anxiously, where were all those things? Mom pointed to a set of cabbage pattern teapots on the table, a nine piece peach tea set, and a few vases. She said disappointedly, "That is all that is left. The whole family has to eat, so we had to pawn them one piece after another."

When I was born, I became the third daughter of the Li family. Actually, before I was born, my parents lost a son and a daughter. Those two were after my first and second older sisters and my older brother. Otherwise I would have three older sisters and two older brothers. That was why my parents regarded me as a pearl in the palm of their hands. In Chinese, we say "you are afraid the pearl will melt if you put her in your mouth and you are afraid the pearl will drop to the ground if you hold her in your hands." The whole family worried something might happen to me. As a result, I became the pearl of the whole family. The year I was born, my second elder sister was twelve.

My father told her not to go to school anymore because she had to take care of me as Dad still had to go to work in the Forbidden City. Mom was helping a Japanese doctor clinic in the center ofBeiping near Wang Fu Jing Street.

My second elder sister acted as though she were my mother all her life. My birthday is the same day as hers according the lunar calendar, May the 19th. We two have been very close in our whole life. There were always endless topics between us. I heard so many stories of our Li family from her. Unfortunately she passed away at the age of 86 in 2019. Otherwise, she would be so happy to read this book.

When Grandpa was alive, the Li family did not have to worry about life, but after he passed away, the family situation went from bad to worse. Dad was born in Beiping on September 21, 1904, a year and a half older than the last emperor Puyi, who was born on February 7, 1906. When Puyi was less than three years old, Guang Xu, the puppet emperor, and Empress Dowager Cixi, his aunt, the real ruler of Qing dynasty, died within 24 hours. China's last emperor, Puyi, ascended the throne when he was less than three years old. (December 12, 1908). My second aunt told me that when my father was about 6 years old, he had a job: holding a small yellow umbrella for Puyi. No wonder Dad was more cautious and serious than the average man.

The Forbidden City, which was full of rules, protocols, and strict disciplines, surrounded by heavily fortified walls, was a place where one could not breath freely. There was an old Chinese saying that: "A companion to the emperor is like the companion of a tiger." Dad should have been youthful and vigorous, but he was bound in an invisible spider's web. Dad was always very serious all his life, not allowing even the slightest mistake. There was not a single greasy spot on the fur coat he wore for 30 years. Neither was there a scratch on his black leather shoes. The tense and terrible living environment made Dad's personality seem too rigid, old-fashioned, and too serious about everything. Everyone in the family seemed to be afraid of him. In my mind, Dad was like a big tree reaching up to the sky, nearly 6 feet tall with broad shoulders, mighty and solemn. His eyes were not big, but they were bright and sharp, and nothing could escape his notice. Dad was always dressed neatly, and stylish.

From a young age, I felt that he was a father who loved his children very much. In the cold winter, Dad came back home by bicycle from the Forbidden City. As soon as he got off his bicycle, he handed Mom a bag which contained my favorite donkey meatballs, fried creaks, sausages, and sugar-coated hawthorns. Dad, Mom, my younger sister, and I sat around the small phoebe table on the bed. Dad tasted his liquor, Er Guo Tou, (I call it Chinese Vodka) and fried peanuts. He not only let Mom take a sip from time to time, but also dipped the chopsticks in the liquor glass and gave my sister and I a taste. This was when I could see the rare smile on Dad's face. His smiling face made my heart blossom. When Dad had a smile on his face, the air in the whole room was relaxed.

In some ways he was extremely tough on us. For example, we were not allowed to bring classmates to our home casually. A visit from a female classmate to the house had to be approved by him. The boys had no chance to visit at all. When Dad was alive, only two female classmates were allowed to come to my house to play with me. When I was growing up, I forgot how many rules my sister and I had to follow. My great school classmate Su Enjuan once joked with me when she said, "Thanks to your father, who disciplined you so strictly, otherwise I could hardly imagine what kind of naughty girl you would grow into."

Since I was a child, the adults worried about me as I always had accidents. For instance, I was easily knocked down by bigger schoolmates, fell off the slide, and the worst thing was that I would faint easily. My second elder sister once told my American husband, "She (referring to me) will never grow up and always make people worry about her. It seems she will be in danger at all times." My American husband also worried about me. He had to do everything himself. When we both went out, he wouldn't let me drive. When I drove myself, he worried until I came home. He wouldn't let me carry the groceries back into the house, for fear that I would fall. I was really pampered.

When I was in the 5th grade in elementary school, my father needed to write his bio to the leader. He asked me to write it. Dad proudly said to me, "Your dad has been this tough guy all his life. He hasn't done anything wrong, and that is why he's not afraid of anything. When the Communist Party established a new China, the government officials gathered all of us who were working in the Forbidden City into the Daoist Temple (Dong Yue Temple) outside the Chaoyang Gate. They asked us questions, mainly to see who had taken anything from the Forbidden City without permission. Over the years, there had always been unclean hands who stole things from the palace. No matter what they asked me, I gave the same answer, 'A man is not afraid of the shadow crooked.' Dad's words had a huge impact on me. Dad's hard-boned personality also let me inherit it. No matter what happened in my life, no matter how much I was wronged, I was never afraid of anybody or give up.

During the Cultural Revolution in 1966, many people

"betrayed" classmates, colleagues, friends, superiors, teachers, and even family members in order to save themselves, or succumbed to various pressures and did something wrong to innocent people. I still had my father's hard-bone character. I was not afraid of anything and dared to stand on the table with the rebels to argue that "When one's father is a hero, his son is a good man; while when one's father is a reactionary bastard, his son is a bad guy" was a fallacy. As a girl, I dared to debate with a group of male rebels in front of the school's library. No matter how much they ridiculed me and laughed at me, I was not afraid and argued with reason. In the end they had to leave. Wherever I went, I was the one who dared to stand out and spoke for justice. I was born a Manchu princess but never enjoy the title. However, the strong character and never bow my head to anybody accompanied me to overcome many obstacles in my life.

In fact, each of us already has a position in the world even before we are born. For example, born in what kind of family, poor or rich, the people you will meet in your life, whether you make friends or enemies, whether you are a lover, or a husband or wife, whether you have harmonious brothers or sisters (including your children) whether they come to repay, or to revenge, whether they come to be friends, or passers-by, all these are predestined and cannot be changed. Whoever you meet in this world is destined. There is evil fate; there is good fate. In short, the people who come into your life all have a purpose and a mission. It is Karma.

Growing up, I was proud that, despite my being delicate and squeamish, God took good care of me. I was doing very well in all disciplines. Actually I didn't put much effort into it. Paying attention and listening to the teachers carefully in class, and understanding quickly, were my ways of keeping myself on top of the class. I also had a good memory and finished my homework right after class. There were no chores for me to do at home, and playing hard, running fast, jumping high, were all I had to do. In the fourth grade of primary school, I didn't know what track and field were, but I was chosen by a P.E. teacher to join the school track and field team. I didn't know what gymnastics was, but at the age of 12 in the first year of junior high school, I was selected by the Beijing Shi Cha Hai Youth Amateur Sports School to practice gymnastics. (Jet Li was training at the same school too). Thanks to the five years of training in that School, it not only cured my bronchitis, but also laid a solid foundation for my exercise habits for the rest of my life.

In addition to sports, I also liked to sing and dance. When I was a teenager, I attended Beijing Chao Yang Men Junior Choir and the Dong Cheng Workers' Club Junior Dance Team. I was elected the leader of the class and I acted like I was really the leader. I was so bold that I took the whole class to climb Jingshan Hill across from the back door of The Palace Museum and to row boats in the lake of Bei Hai Park. I had never studied music, but when the class needed a singing conductor, the teacher asked me to try and I did it. All these activities had trained me to be brave, confident, and good at organizing social events. Not only I was good at it, but I also had a lot of fun with it. I've benefited all my life from these opportunities. I was deeply grateful to the teachers, coaches and classmates who gave me these opportunities and nurtured me.

My life was happy and carefree. Under the cultivation of my teachers, under the care of my parents, brothers and sisters, and under the company of my younger sister who was never jealous but supported me, I was like a flower bathed in the sunshine and rain of love, thriving and living happily through my childhood.

Chapter 3

My Youth

When I was 12 years old, I graduated from Chao Yang Men Primary School in Dong Cheng District, Beijing, and was admitted to Beijing No. 23 Middle School with a score of 100 points in mathematics and 85 points in Chinese. Probably because my score had already exceeded the score line to be admitted to the school, on the first day, schoolteacher Huang announced that I was appointed to be the class monitor. I was flattered and functioned as the leader of the class.

Five years of gymnastics spare time training at Shi Cha Hai Sports School from 12 to 17 years old had turned me into a strong-willed girl with athlete's physique and endurance. After I broke my right elbow jumping off the balance beam from a handstand position without the coach on site, I still practiced handstands with my left hand while my right arm was wrapped with a splint! Because of the good sports environment in Shi Cha Hai Amateur Sports School, I also learned how to swim and skate by myself.

Besides this athletic ability, at school I was a straight-A student. This had had both a positive and negative impact on my personality throughout my life. In face of difficulties, I would not get discouraged or bow my head. I never gave up until I reached my goal. My self-confidence was extremely strong. I was very competitive, and always strived to be the best. Earlier I talked about the pampering from my family, especially my parents and my second elder sister, who regarded me as a pearl in the palm of their hands. One the other hand, my squeamish and prideful character had always followed me.

Everything, like a coin, has two sides. I also have several incomprehensible weaknesses. First of all, I am afraid of insects and animals. In junior high school at second year of chemistry class, there was a class studying the anatomy of a frog. Most of the students were very curious and excited. But I didn't dare to go into the laboratory. The teacher said to me, "If you cannot do it, you can still watch others do it." I didn't even dare to look at the frog, let alone to see it dissected, so I simply stood outside the lab for a whole period. Teacher Wu was very unhappy, but there was nothing I could do about it. Later, when I grew up, I found that my mother and sisters were actually similar to me: neither of them could pick up a cat or a dog. After arriving in the United States, I often made a scene when there were dogs or cats around me. The most interesting phenomenon is I don't know why cats and dogs liked to pounce on me. Americans treat cats and dogs as pets, so they cannot not understand how and why I am so hysterical when animals come near me.

Secondly, my body cannot tolerate cold or heat. Once in a winter physical class, everyone had to stand in the playground listening to the teacher's lecture. My hands and feet were sore from the cold that I cried. When the teacher found out and asked me what had happened, I cried and said, 'Tm too cold." The physical education teacher didn't know whether to cry or laugh.

As the monitor of the class, I was crying just because I was too cold! He said, "Then go into the classroom. You don't need to cry for such a little thing."

From the first year of junior high school to the third year, from twelve to fifteen years old, my personality traits were also formed during this period. I was like a blossoming thorny rose, a galloping pony, a newborn calf that was not afraid of tigers, a bird that had just grown feathers. All in all, I spent three years of junior high school happily and carefree.

It was soon time to apply for high school or vocational school. Another classmate, Geng Xiuqi and I, were selected to skip the exam and were awarded to go to a normal school. Not only was there no tuition, room and board were also free. I went home and happily told my parents. Unexpectedly, when Dad heard it, his face darkened and he said, "Have you heard the old saying: if a family has two buckets of grain, no one in the family would become the king of children!" Dad's reaction rejected the offer by the school.

However, I needed to make an application for high school, but to which school? Mom, Dad and I couldn't make up our minds. Teacher Huang, who taught us Russian lessons, had always appreciated my bravery and fluency in speaking Russian, so he suggested that I apply for the Preparatory Course of Beijing Foreign Trade Institute. I liked foreign languages very much, and more importantly, the school was near the old Gulou Street (Drum Tower), which was very close to my home. I applied. After being admitted, I was assigned to study English. I was disappointed, because the school also had Russian classes. I would love to continue learning Russian. However, in those days, students didn't have the freedom to choose what they wanted to learn. Everything was assigned. In fact, learning English proved to be very useful later.

At that time, to be accepted by a high school was a big event. On the day I move to the school, my father, mother, second elder sister, her husband, my younger sister, and Xiaoying, the first granddaughter of the Li family, all turned out to accompanied me to the Preparatory

Course of the Foreign Trade Institute. All the girls were assigned to live on the third floor of the red building. The boys lived on the first and second floors. Some students also had parents to accompany them to school, but my whole family, three generations, all accompanied me to school. My schoolmates all looked at me with envious eyes. I felt I'd grown up. Immersing myself in the happiness of love, I made up my mind to study hard and honor my ancestors for the Li family. These three years of preparatory courses that life had laid before me gave me a solid foundation for my future life, and some of my school mates have become my life-long friends.

According to the school regulations, no matter where your home was, everyone had to live in the school. You were allowed to go home after class only on Saturday afternoons, but had to come back to school for evening study before 7 p.m. on Sundays. Three meals a day had to be eaten in the canteen according to your assigned table.

At 6 o'clock in the morning, as soon as the radio loudspeaker sounded, we had to get up immediately to run to Lake Houhai. I was the platoon leader of the girls, shouting slogans to lead everyone to run around or make a half circle of the lake. After running, one could stay by the lake to read foreign language books and then come back to school for breakfast. We had four classes in the morning, three classes in the afternoon, English, Chinese, mathematics, geometry, physics, history, politics, chemistry and sports. In the afternoon after class, everyone had to go to the large playground of Xiao Shi Qiao street where the Teacher's dormitory was located, to participate in various sports: basketball, volleyball, martial arts, running, high jump, long jump and so on. My home is also in Xiao Shi Qiao street, once a while I sneaked home to have a bite given by my mom.

Our Preparatory Course at the Foreign Trade Institute was a school under the Ministry of Foreign Trade, and the Ministry had its own farm. The cafeterias of our school were provided with better food, and from time to time there were meats such as lamb, pork, large shrimps and so on. At the beginning of 1960s China had a famine and most of us were 16 to 19 years old, which was still the time to grow, and we needed that nutrition. Thanks to the care of the Ministry of Foreign Trade, we all grew up healthy.

On September 1, 1964, I proudly walked into the doors of the university. That pride is still unforgettable. There were thirteen English classes, two Japanese classes, and four French classes. The first three classes of English were students who came from the Preparatory Course. According to my score, I was placed in the first class of English, and that was the top class. Since then, hard work and hard competition had also become the goal of each of us. How I wish life would all be smooth sailing! However, life is just a bitter sea. Every one of us has to experience "life" before crossing to the other side.

Chapter 4

Unforgettable College Life

Our English class was the smallest of the thirteen English classes, with a total of sixteen students, eight males and eight females. Director Miao Junqing of the school and several other teachers selected the committees for each class. I was appointed a member of the class committee in charge of physical education and recreational activities.

The teachers assigned to teach our class had the strongest academic background. Mr. Zhang Yinyu (Charlie Chang) in charge of our English writing class, graduated from Cambridge University in the United Kingdom. Liang Xianzhang, a descendant of overseas Chinese in the United States, was in charge of listening and speaking classes. The respected Provost Mr. Li Dezi sometimes taught us English Rhetoric.

In later days we heard about our teachers' family background. Mr. Zhang Yinyu's father was Zhang Tiesheng, a tycoon in the field of Shanghai textile industry who had gone to Hong Kong before the Communist took over China. Vice Premier Chen Yi personally sent a telegram to invite Mr. Zhang Tiesheng to come back to mainland China, but he refused. It turned out to be a troublesome family background for his son, my beloved teacher, Zhang Yinyu later.

Mr. Liang's father was the editor-in-chief of an English language newspaper in Hong Kong. Although Mr. Liang had never studied abroad, his mother was an overseas Chinese in Hawaii, so he spoke authentic American English since his childhood. Our sixteen uniquely gifted students have since then begun our unforgettable university competitive life.

September 18t, 1964, was the first day of our class of English. Mr. Zhang Yinyu wore an ironed blue suit. He was medium height, thin in stature, wearing a pair of black-rimmed glasses, and carried a black briefcase under his right arm. He looked graceful and handsome. From head to toe, he was full of the shrewdness of Shanghainese, and the talent and demeanor of returning scholars from the Great Britain. Mr. Zhang looked very excited, almost like a child jumped onto the podium of the classroom. It took me many years later to understand why he was so energized and excited that day.

Mr. Zhang was born in a large family in Jiangsu province. His father went to Hong Kong before New China was established in 1949. He sent his two sons to study in the great Britain before 1949. Mr. Zhang Yinyu and his brother passed through Hong Kong on the way back from England to see their father. He did not listen to their father's advice not to return to mainland China and returned to Shanghai with the persuasion of his eldest brother,. Mr. Zhang Yinyu later regretted that decision but it was too late. He later told me he graduated from a mission high school in Shanghai and was sent to study in the Great Britain. He originally selected English literature, studying Shakespeare in Cambridge. His father was very angry after he heard his son studied Shakespeare. "Why not learn a useful engineering subject?" So Mr. Zhang was forced to transfer to the Printing Institute in the Great Britain to study printing. After returning to China, he was depressed, but after all, he was an intellectual who returned to China and had a diploma from an English printing school, so he was assigned to work in Bank of China as a senior engineer.

Unfortunately, In 1957, Mr. Zhang was labelled as a rightist and exiled to Inner Mongolia for years to look after cows. Later he was sent to carry stones in a mine in Shandong province. God's care, and his tenacious vitality, not only allowed him to escape death on several occasions, but also gave him a strong body, hard as iron. His strong body and his steeled will helped him survive the labor camp and the Cultural Revolution. After more than ten years of torture, he was told to teach his beloved English at a first-class foreign language university in Beijing. That is my university, Beijing Foreign Trade Institute, now a prestigious University named The University of International Business and Economics, on par with Peking University and Tsinghua University. How could he not be excited? The details of his experience will be told later.

In the sixties, we rarely saw a teacher in a suit at school. What was even more surprising was that when he came to the podium, he spoke English not a word of Chinese. Although we were all highly qualified students who had already studied English for three years in the Preparatory Course, we rarely listened to live English lectures and we were all confused. However, Mr. Zhang didn't seem to notice it. After a class, we felt like we had been traveling in clouds and walking through mountain fog. It was this rigorous and immersive training that turned us into English-speaking college students in a few months.

Another teacher I must speak of is Liang Xianzhang. As I mentioned above, I heard that his father was the English editor of the Hong Kong Ta Kung Pao and his mother was an American overseas Chinese in Hawaii, who spoke American English to him since his childhood. His sister worked at VOA. Mr. Liang never went abroad but grew up speaking American English and later went to the English Department of Beijing Normal University. After graduating from that university, he was assigned to teach in a city in Hebei Province. In 1964, he was transferred to our school to teach us oral English. Teacher Liang's method was also emphasize listening and speaking. First: We listened to the news in English repeatedly without seeing an English word. Then he either asked questions for us to answer or let us retell the news in English.

I remembered a few times one or two female classmates of mine were not able to answer questions and were in tears. I, a young woman who loved to be challenged, found the joy of learning in this class. Whenever I could understand the news, my heart was full of joy and I bravely raised my hand to answer the teacher's questions. As a result, I had more chances to speak English in class and my confidence became stronger and stronger. It laid a good foundation for me to be able to deliver my thoughts and speak in public later in my life. Now I became a grandma, I trained my granddaughter to act as a journalist when she was only 7 years old and videotaped her at the same time. I asked several questions and she took so much joy to answer me. Not only we had a lot of fun watching the videotape, she had built up her speaking abilities and confidence.

For early morning runs, I loved the tranquil Lake Houhai and the weeping willows along the shore. I always stayed there reading or memorizing my favorite English stories. Then I came back to school to wash myself, go to the cafeteria for breakfast, and then be in the classroom at eight o'clock.

We had four classes in the morning and three in the afternoon. These seven lessons are all in English, either intensive reading of things like news, or listening and oral practice. Sometimes we had Linguaphone style for pronunciation & intonation exercises. In the afternoon after class, everyone had to go to the playground to do exercise, also known as Physical Education class. We played basketball, volleyball, or practiced martial arts before running. After eating dinner at six o'clock, we started self-study in the classroom from seven to nine o'clock. At ten o'clock the lights in the dorm must turn out and everyone went to bed. We were living like soldiers every day, with a military discipline, and there was not enough free time, but no one complained. On the contrary, everyone was working very hard, and we also helped each other in every way. English was the center of our lives and bound us together. Sixteen of us were fortunate enough to have two high-level teachers teaching us to speak and write English. We sprung up like mushrooms.

As we made a big progress in our English study, sometimes teachers from other classes or schools came over to listen to our classes, which were called big open classes. Teacher Zhang was always very excited and nervous. We did our best to make him feel good and proud of his teaching. He watched us study hard, actively cooperating with his teaching. His heart was full of joy. I was full of energy every day. The pain of the passing away of my father had slowly left me after three years. The love of my mother and sisters and the joy of my new life at the university also made me slowly adapt to life without my father.

I was both a member of the cultural arts and sports committees, and a member of the Youth League branch. All teachers liked me, classmates loved me. I was like a butterfly falling into a honeypot. Learning and playing were my two tasks. It was also a great pleasure to sneak home every other day to see my mother and my nieces and nephews. But the good times were short-lived. In the third year of college, the Cultural Revolution broke out in China.

Chapter 5

The Cultural Revolution

I remembered it was early June 1966. As usual, the school's loudspeaker sounded on time, but the particularly serious tone of the broadcaster brought everyone to a halt. It turned out that Nie Yuanzi and some others at Beijing University posted a large character poster criticizing the leadership of the school's party committee. The Central People's Broadcast Station repeated from time to time the entire contents of this big-character poster. Students who were concerned and sensitive to politics immediately understood what this was all about because in the past few months, the People's Daily had published a series of large articles criticizing the "Three Men Village", Deng Tuo, Wu Han, Liao Mo-sha. Yao Wen-yuan's article criticized a play written by Wu Han, "Hai Rui's Dismissal," as an example of anti Communist sentiment.

Although I was twenty years old, I was still like an innocent and nai:ve girl. First of all, I was not very concerned with politics. Secondly, I did not believe there were any contradictions within the Communist Party. I was only interested in learning English. Suddenly the whole school was like ants on a hot pot! Students were running around but nobody went to the classroom. Some students got together to talk about what was happening and some even found newspapers, taking brushes and ink to write their own big-character posters. I was very lost and disappointed. I asked loudly, "Why is it so messy? Why not go to the classroom to start class?" A classmate scolded me disapprovingly, "Didn't you see what had happened? You still want to go to class to study?"

At eight o'clock, when the teachers came to the school for classes, no one said a word. The whole school had become a boiling pot of porridge. In less than two hours, a large poster questioning the party committee of the Institute of Foreign Trade was also posted. Party secretary Yang Ruidian was also publicly criticized. Later, inexplicable accusations such as "Wrong educational line," or "School of revisionism" were aiming at the leadership of the school. The quiet campus became an uncontrollable political battlefield. The students naturally divided into two factions-the rebels and the royalists or conservatives.

Those who wrote big-character posters to expose their teachers had become rebels. Most of the students' leaders, and those who did not agree with the views of the rebels, were called royalists. Both factions later formed their own Red Guards organizations. Writing big posters against each other and debating political issues that they themselves were not clear about became daily life. In short, my dream of becoming a translator was put aside. The sixteen highly achieving students in our English class, who had been directly selected from the preparatory course, had loved each other, helped each other, and got along well, now suddenly became two hostile factions. Seven male and two female students became rebels. Six others including me , plus one man, were called hardcore, steel royalists. The whole school became a sea of big character posters.

I couldn't understand why our school had suddenly implemented a revisionist educational line, the white capitalist road, and how we could become the seedlings of revisionism. Big-character posters attacking individuals also appeared, one after another. Although my family was Manchu, the so-called nobility, I was not criticized. In 1911, the revolutionaries headed by Dr. Sun Yetsen abolished the Qing Dynasty ruled by Manchus. Before new China was established in 1949, my father worked as a curator in the Forbidden City. He was considered a worker, besides, our family didn't own any private properties, neither did we have relatives living abroad (families who had relatives living abroad were accused of being spies.)

Personally, I was impeccable in every aspect, but I was still "exposed" one day in big characters. (Chatting with my sister, who was thousands of miles away from me on WeChat while I was writing this autobiography, she mentioned that during the Cultural Revolution, when she went to my school to look for me. Before she could enter the school, she saw a big sign posted on the school gate: "Down with the hardcore traitor Li Chongjun, a revisionist seedling!" That was the name I went by while in school! I don't remember much about the incident, only remembered that my name appeared on a big character poster, criticizing me because I did not do any chores at home. It was saying that I was spoiled rotten even my handkerchief was washed by my mother. I was very embarrassed after reading it. I thought "that was my mother's love for me. What does it have to do with you?" Anyway, no one in the whole school dared to learn English at that time. Classes were all cancelled. Everyone either went outside of the school to read the big-character posters in other schools, or wrote their own big character posters every day. The whole society had changed. Many leaders were labeled: "Taking the capitalist road." People with problematic family backgrounds, including those who had overseas relations, those who have participated in the Kuomintang earlier, those who had houses and land in their families, and even primary and secondary school teachers who were usually active in their work and were conscientious and responsible, had all become the targets of the revolution. Any student had the right to go to the teacher's house and "raid the house" at will. Insults, teasing, torturing teachers, forcing them to wear tall hats, hanging big signs around their necks, punishing them to their knees, beating them, shaving their hair into a yin-yang symbol (with one half bald), happened every day. The Great Proletarian Cultural Revolution provided many people with the opportunity to vent their personal anger and revenge on those whom they disliked in the past.

My mood grew more and more depressed each day. I was hoping and looking forward to the end of this chaotic social life. But contrary to my expectation, on August 5, 1966, the People's Daily, the Central People's Broadcast Station published "My Big Character Poster" written by Mao Ze-dong, the most prominent leader in China. The rebels cheered and jumped after listening to it. After I listened to it, my heart sank, and my hopes flagged. I realized that this revolution would not end soon at all but was just starting. I didn't know when I would ever be able to learn English again.

On August 18, 1966, Mao Zedong received the Red Guards at the Tiananmen Tower. Both factions in our school set up their own Red Guards organizations. Neither of them obeyed the other, and they all went to Tiananmen Square. I also followed the crowds. In the distance, I saw the tall figure of Mao Ze-dong waving to people and many people were so excited that they cried, but I couldn't get excited. My heart was dark and sullen. After returning to school, I did not go back to school. My felt depressed and I couldn't stand the atmosphere in the school, so I took time to go home to visit my mother and played with my nephews and nieces.

The children's sweet little faces, and their innocent hearts always gave me infinite joy. Playing with them helped me forget all the pains in the world. I've been like this for years and I love being with kids. Later, I went abroad, traveled around the world, and became a grandma. The greatest joy in the world was with my grandson Aaron and my granddaughter Audrey. Even when I was about 70, I still did somersaults on the carpet with them. Everyone said I didn't act like an adult, but I couldn't explain it myself. The joy of playing with them was something that no amount of money could buy. Their energy and happiness mood lifted me. Vise versa, as a grown up, my sincerity to be their playmate and happy laughter also made them like me even more. Perhaps this child's heart of mine suffered too much in the cruelty of social life. I trusted people easily, believed what people said and easily spoke out what was in my mind. I never consider the consequences of speaking the truth. This "simplicity" or innocence often led me into trouble. But I never regretted it. Wherever I go, I have friends who like me. It is easy to cultivate a mountain, but it is difficult to change one's character, and build a new mountain. Maybe this character of mine will follow me to another world.

The flames of the Cultural Revolution had been burning, wave after wave. Every morning, reading Mao's words in the party newspaper became a formality. There was also little communication between the two factions. In addition to Beijing, the Cultural Revolution in other provinces and cities across the country started to fight in great force.

Ningxia Second Beijing Opera Troupe, where my second elder sister and her husband worked, also clearly divided into two factions. They were the same two terms: One faction called themselves the revolutionary rebels and the other group were being called royalists (conservatives). There were only about eighty people in the whole Peking opera Troup and of these, only eight were conservatives. My second elder sister and her husband were two of those eight. My brother-in-law was just an ordinary actor and the head of the Human

Resources Section, working diligently every day. However, he was given a name, called "the capitalist roader," and was dragged into the streets to be paraded and punished, then forced to kneel. Fortunately he was not beaten. Later the Peking Opera Troupe rebels and some rebels in the community united to start more fighting. My sister and her husband immediately left Shi Zui Shan where they were assigned to work and returned to Beijing. My mom and I were very happy to see them. At that time, everyone was issued a coupon to buy groceries. However, after a long time, the monthly salary and grain coupon of my sister and her husband were cut off. Their son Xiao Chun and daughter Jingjing, plus Mom and I, the family of six, were all going to have problems.

My brother-in-law who had never asked for help all his life, had to write a letter to his colleagues and old friends in Yinchuan asking for help. Soon, he received two hundred yuan and a grocery coupon worth two hundred pounds from Ru Shaokui and his wife, Yan Baojun as well Cheng Yanqiu's eldest disciple, Mr. Wang Yinqiu, also sent three hundred yuan. What gracious generosity this was! Our family never forgot that they helped us through that difficult situation.

It was at this time, when the future was so uncertain, that my Tai Chi practice was improving. My second elder sister and her husband were forced to leave their home and did not know what would happen next. They were in a bad mood. My second elder sister somehow learned that a Tai Chi teacher taught Tai Chi at Lake Houhai very early every morning. She asked me to accompany her. I hated getting up early, but in order to accompany my dear sister, I struggled to get up at 5 a.m. The teacher seemed to be seventy or eighty years old, tall and thin, with a straight body, even his hair had not turned grey. I didn't know who he was. Seven or eight people came each day. He led everyone in the practice of twenty-four styles of Tai Chi movements from 5:30 to 6:30 a.m. No one talked and people left right after the practice was over. I was the only young girl among them. The teacher said my movements were too undulating and personally demonstrated it to me.

When he practiced Tai Chi, he was like a mountain. His firm gaze seemed to be able to see through everything, but his movements were like floating clouds and flowing water, smooth and elegant. His guidance laid a good foundation for me to teach Tai Chi later. In those dark times, on the shores of that dark Lake Houhai, he gave me a power that words could not express. Tai Chi helped me overcome depression and loneliness in my later life many times. Through the practice of Tai Chi, I accepted the energy from the universe, opened up the blocked meridians, and opened a new realm in my heart. To the unknown old Tai Chi teacher, who showed me how to Tai Chi, I have to bow deeply to the sky, believing that we will meet again in another world.

The Cultural Revolution was a touchstone. Everyone's true nature was exposed to the daylight in this abrasive environment. Good or evil, Yin or Yang, black or white, it was all there with nowhere to hide. How many people lost their innocent lives during the Cultural Revolution? How many people suffered unimaginable insults? How many great and accomplished artists had been persecuted to death! It's unbelievable that so many people betrayed their own colleagues, their friends, their own superiors, their teachers, and their own family members. In fact, this was all the evil consequence of politics.

From then on, I was extremely uninterested in politics, because once you fell into it, it was like taking poison and smoking marijuana! You cannot get rid of it! I was so disheartened by it. What one thinks, says, or does were all controlled by politics! What's even more frightening is that most people don't even dare to think. They couldn't think with their own brains. It seems that one could only remain safe by keeping silent and closing their eyes. How suffocating! I could not stand it!

The situation in the whole country was chaotic. Every province and city seemed to be divided into two factions. Forceful fighting was in full swing, and some rebels even used guns. Posters were flying everywhere and no one knew which was right and which was wrong.

Most of the students became vagrant Peripatetics. I didn't know who suggested it, but our entire department in the city near my home was moved to the west suburbs of Beijing. Every morning, I went to the classroom as required to study Mao Zedong' works with everyone else, but I looked forward to going to the canteen for lunch at noon, and then going back to the dormitory to take a nap. In the afternoon we could do whatever we wished. That was considered our free time. I didn't know when many students began to read the literature books written by western writers. The first time I heard about it was with the book Jane Eyre. Moving from the city to the suburbs also facilitated my contacts with a few girlfriends I knew in my preparatory course years. For me, taking a nap, going for a swim in the canal, or sneaking back home to see my mom and kids were the happiest times.

A very small number of teachers became supporters of the rebels but most of the teachers became the targets of the rebel dictatorship. They were kept in schools and called bulls, ghosts, and snakes. They were often criticized by students. I could not stand to see that the teachers, who were respectable and knowledgeable, were now prisoners. I also couldn't stand to see that the crazy students who got their knowledge from their teachers seemed to have changed their human nature. So I always found excuses not to participate in any meeting criticizing the teachers. I often went home and no one asked me about it.

What I will never forget was one meeting where we were told that everyone had to attend. No one could be absent. I and five other female classmates in our class nervously came to the balcony on the top of our classroom building. The atmosphere that day was very tense. We set at the seats in the last row. I thought to myself: if something happens that I couldn't tolerate, I'll leave the scene.

With a shout from the person who was in charge of the criticism meeting, more than a dozen teachers were brought up. Teacher Zhang Yinyu, who taught our class was also among them. One by one they bowed their heads and stood in the front. There were boards with written characters hanging from their necks. I didn't have the heart to look at what was written on the board. My heart ached. Although thousands of people during the Cultural Revolution were beaten, humiliated, and even killed, this was the first time I had seen with my own eyes the insults to the teachers who had such prestige in the past, and gave us so much knowledge.

I couldn't listen to the speakers at all. I couldn't remember what they were saying. I just remembered a student started to slap the teacher's face. His actions shocked the audience but not even one person stopped him. On the contrary, several students stepped forward and began to imitate him. Although I couldn't see clearly in the last row, I couldn't bear it anymore and left the scene in anger.

I thought at the time, I had no overseas relations (It was a crime if one had relatives who lived abroad, especially in the U.S., Hongkong, Macao or Taiwan). In my family there was nothing wrong which could be used as an excuse to be accused. I had nothing to be afraid oft If someone asked me why I left the meeting, I would say, "I suddenly felt ill, I had to leave." See what you can do!

I went back to my dorm, fidgeting. My heart was filled with pain and sadness. Without telling anyone, I simply left this filthy place. From the western suburbs, I rode my bike back to my home in the city. I took my nieces and nephews to Lake Houhai for a few hours to calm down. I was going to stay at home for a few days when no one would be able to control anyone and no one would have to ask anyone for leave. If anyone pressed me, I would say I was sick. Because when I was in school, although I was good in sports, I appeared very vulnerable in health. My body was squeamish. I would get sick when the weather was too hot or too cold. Every semester when we were sent to do manual labor, everyone would take care of me and gave me the lightest work. Even then when we came back to school I was often sick.

One winter in the first year of college, I came back from digging a canal at the Agricultural University. Everyone else was fine but I had a high fever and the doctor admitted me to the Drum Tower Hospital for unknown reasons. The whole class came to the hospital to visit me. So now being so sick that I couldn't go to school was the best excuse I had to stay at home at the time. The 16 students in our class were divided into two factions. After all, we grew up together in Beijing. Since entering the university, eating, living, studying, and exercising, we were always together. I was a popular student. I was sure they would not do anything to me. I stayed at home for one night and was still reluctant to go back to school. The scene of the meeting and beating teachers at school yesterday was still vividly in my mind and torturing me.

The second day I planned to go to the grocery store on Drum Tower Street to buy something after lunch. Just as I stepped out the gate of our yard, I saw a person in a short distance pushing a coal cart. Generally it was rare to see people push such a coal cart on the road. The man pushing the cart wore thick glasses. Isn't that Teacher Zhang

Yinyu? I made up my mind that I would come up to greet him and call him Teacher Zhang loudly.

It should have been a consolation for him when he would hear his student greet him. We were walking towards each other, getting closer and closer. I was about to go up and greet him, but he seemed to deliberately not see me, as if ashamed. He quickly turned his head and pushed the cart forward. In that instant, I saw that his cheeks under his glasses were not only black and purple but also swollen. What happened? Why did he see me walking toward him and deliberately dodge away? I stood dumbfounded in the street. For the first time in my life I saw a person's face so swollen and dark purple with bruises! Could it be that he was slapped yesterday after I left the scene of the criticism meeting? Wouldn't he want to hear his distressed students greet him as a teacher now?

For many years, I still can't forget the awkward and terrible shock of that encounter. More than twenty years later, he came to visit my home in the United States. Several times I wanted to mention that encounter but I couldn't. Let the heavy stone sink in my heart forever, I thought.

When I was in Italy writing my autobiography, I talked to my Italian neighbor about this, saying I didn't understand why my teacher turned his head away. Her husband said that he was trying to protect me. How come I did not understand that Teacher Zhang was afraid of causing me trouble, and that was why he ignored me? Decades later I found the answer from a foreigner who had never been to China! My heart was so sad. Teacher Zhang had passed away. I wanted to give him a hug.

I don't know when the big tantrum suddenly became hot everywhere. The country's college, middle and primary school students could take a train or car to go anywhere without buying a ticket, and wherever they went, there were reception teams to arrange their lodging including free food. Students in Beijing were pouring out of the city. Many students formed various groups and walked to Yan'an, Jing Gang Shan, Hunan and other old revolutionary base areas. I didn't have the courage and physical strength to join them. The school was basically empty, and all the students from other places came to live there. I heard that the big tantrum would soon stop. Two female classmates and I decided to take the train to Guangzhou. Because the twice a-year Guangzhou Trade Fair would be the place where we practiced English, but the Cultural Revolution didn't even have classes. How could there be any opportunity to go to Guangzhou for an internship?

The three of us arrived at Beijing Railway Station. It was crowded with people but it was easy to find the train to Guangzhou. However, we could not get close enough to board the train at all. If we lost this opportunity, we would never have the chance to go visit that charming city. We three decided to give it a try. We all held hands and pressed towards the nearest carriage with many others. The seats were already full of people, but we flocked into the luggage compartment and many others. It was a carriage without seats. Should we try? I said, let's get on! So the three of us squeezed into the luggage compartment. There were no seats, no toilets, and everyone was sitting on the floor.

Soon, the floor of the carriage was full of people, but here were more people still squeezing in. "Close the door!" Someone shouted. It was hot and stuffy. We were all looking forward to an early departure. I couldn't remember how long it took for the train to finally leave the Beijing Railway Station with overwhelmed students who were completely lost.

After three days and three nights, our train arrived in Guang Zhou. Along the way, as soon as the train stopped, we were busy looking for toilets and trying to find food peddlers on the platform. After the train entered Hunan province, the door was opened. At long last we could breathe some fresh air. That was the first time I saw the landscape of the South with my own eyes. I don't know why I have loved the scenery of the south since I was a child: the pavilions, the small bridges, the flowing water, the green fields and the red soil made me feel relaxed and comfortable. There is always a sweet smell of the south in my heart. More than twenty years later, I met Mr. Yang who had been the director and photographer of Beijing People's Art Theater Group and had practiced Buddhism for more than twenty years.

When talking about my past life, he told me that during the Qing Dynasty I was the daughter of a rich tea merchant in the south. He told me that I liked piano, chess, calligraphy, painting, and Taoism. Mr. Yang also said that you could find traces of past lives in your real life now. No wonder when I was young, as soon as I entered the Summer Palace, I went straight to Xie Qu Garden (a beautiful garden imitating the landscape and scenery of the south). Every time I went there, I was reluctant to leave. Later, when I worked at different places, I visited Suzhou, Hangzhou Wuxi, Ningbo, Nanjing and Zhenjiang. I was always lingering in the south. Mr. Yang also told me, "During the Song Dynasty, I couldn't find you in China. It was the Renaissance time." Curiously, I asked him, "So where was I?" He said, "You were in Italy." I was half-convinced but as the Song Dynasty was 960 to 1279, I realized he must be speaking about my past lives.

Later, after studying Buddhism, I have learned that a person's past life will leave deep traces in one's present life. It is almost impossible to get rid of that karma. Believe it or not, Fate is Fate. One cannot change it whatsoever. The only change one can do is to change your way of thinking or your attitude.

Let's go back to the time of the Cultural Revolution. When we arrived in Guangzhou, we were greeted and sent by the local Red Guards to the South China Normal University. On the streets of Guangzhou, there were flowers everywhere and green grass. We had never seen such tall trees with red flowers. Although it was autumn, it felt like summer. All three of us were labeled as conservative royalists at the beginning of the Cultural Revolution. Now no one knew our background or any details of our lives. This anonymity was a saving grace! We took the bus free to go read the big-character posters in various schools. We also climbed the Bai Yun mountain. I can't forget the uncomfortable experience of sleeping on the floor every day, and I don't want to repeat it. After nearly a month of traveling I had very little money in my pocket. I also worried that my mother was concerned about me. We went back to Beijing.

It was early winter in Beijing. We just returned from the sunny south and Beijing not only had cool temperatures but a gloomy atmosphere enveloped the whole city and it was suffocating. The school seemed deserted. No one had smile on their face and no one spoke. The air was heavy and stale. Both the weather and our hearts were cloudy, sullen, and dark.

I didn't know what waited for us. When I went back to the school dormitory, the rest of my classmates also came back from the big tantrum. Some walked to Yan'an and some took the train to Xi'an. I had nothing to do every day. I did not dare to learn English because the classes had stopped. Whoever dared to learn a foreign language might run the risk of being labeled as taking the road of a capitalist and revisionist. Wearing this heavy "hat" was like carrying a big black cauldron on your back and being unable to lift your head.

All kinds of tabloids littered society, and posters were everywhere. People in each province, city, county, and region were divided into two factions. They were all taking resounding names, such as Xiangjiang Wind and Thunder, Revolutionary Storm, Death Squad and so on. Armed struggles became common throughout the country, and armies also participated in local organizations everywhere. In those days, being arrested, beaten, and killed became common happenings. Where was the dignity of an individual? Human life was not worth anything in this period!

From the summer of 1966 to 1968, the country was in turmoil. Today this one was pulled out, and tomorrow that one was criticized. Even those darlings of the beginning of the revolution, those rebels, suddenly became some kind of "linkage" elements, "5.16" elements. (May 16 was the day of the first major political declaration of the Cultural Revolution and summarized Mao's justifications for the Cultural Revolution.) They became targets for arrest and many were repudiated. There was no standard for who was right or wrong.

The order from above was called "Going back to Classrooms and Making Revolution." At least it brought us back to the classroom. Teacher Zhang also returned. He was much "quieter." The only thing that hadn't changed was his passion for English and his seriousness in teaching. According to the study schedule before the Cultural Revolution, he was supposed to teach us the works of the great British writer Shakespeare. Now all the teaching materials became the English version of Mao's three articles. Years later when I mentioned this change of teaching materials for our English class, the listeners all laughed Speaking of Shakespeare, I can never forget the story. As I mentioned earlier, Mr. Zhang Tiesheng, the father of my Teacher Zhang Yinyu, was born in Jiangsu and became a well-known textile tycoon in Shanghai. He sent his two sons, Mr. Zhang and his elder brother to a school taught in English from an early age; and later sent them to The Great Britain to study. Mr. Zhang Yinyu was admitted to the famous Cambridge University. His father originally let him study engineering, but as soon as Teacher Zhang came into contact with Shakespeare's works, he was deeply attracted by the language, humor and plot of this world-famous writer. Like a sponge, he sucked in the talent of this great British literary master and was able to recite Shakespeare's plays and verses in whole paragraphs.

"To be, or not to be, that is the question...." When Mr. Zhang recited this famous verse of the Danish prince in the third act of Shakespeare's Hamlet with an authentic London accent, I was deeply moved. That's why I later took two semesters of Shakespeare classes when I studied for my master's degrees. I also went to Ashland City in Oregon to watch Shakespeare plays several times. To begin with, I was influenced by Teacher Zhang. Secondly, I wanted to make his dream come true through me. The third reason was Shakespeare's characters were like the characters in the famous Chinese novel, A Dream of Red Mansions. There were more than four hundred characters in the novel, all vivid, no similarities. I was so fascinated by Shakespeare' s works.

Please allow me to jump ahead in time. After I came to the U.S. I went to Humboldt State University of California to study for a master's degree in English and American Literature. The director in charge of graduate studies was Professor Turner. He was an expert in the study of Shakespeare. Because he was not sure of my English level even though according to the diploma of the Institute of Beijing Foreign Trade, my transcripts of good scores and three letters of recommendation plus an interview, he accepted my application, but he told me there was a condition : I needed to take three courses for undergraduate students in the English department. After one semester he then would decide whether to accept me as a graduate student in the English department. I signed up for his Shakespeare class.

A few years later, he wrote me a letter of recommendation as a Ph.D. candidate, and he said, "The English Department of our university has never accepted any students who came from the Chinese mainland to enroll in our English Department, let alone graduate studies. Lydia is an exception. I asked her to take three undergraduate courses before I made a final decision, but I didn't expect how quickly she would prove that her English proficiency, expressiveness and comprehension skills far exceeded our expectations."

In fact, when I took Professor Turner's Shakespeare's class, I encountered great challenges. Of course, the influence of Teacher Zhang Yinyu was one of the important driving forces. I had also seen Shakespeare's play Measure for Measure performed by the Master Yu Shizhi of Beijing People's Art Theatre, and Othello performed by Tan Yuanyuan, a major leading ballet dancer in the San Francisco Ballet Troup. Shakespeare's fascinating plot, ingenious conception, and sharp language, drew me into an incredible world of literature. I cherished this learning opportunity very much. However, Shakespeare's works were all written in original ancient English. Even if I knew the plot of the story, it read like a book in heaven.

Fortunately, the school library had every version of Shakespeare's films, as well as a recordings by actors. I took the original text and looked at the movie or listened to the recordings. The old English language suddenly came alive. I could not only understand it but also enjoyed the clever connections and the humor of the language. Each individual character became alive. Because I was fully prepared, it was much easier to take Professor Turner's Shakespeare class. I could quickly find the examples he gave and the original quotes. In particular, his analysis of the characters and plot fascinated me. He occasionally asked questions to test whether we had read or understood. Few people in class could answer his questions. I was the oldest in the class. My life experience was the most abundant. I could see the teacher's satisfying smile and the surprising looks from the students when I expressed my opinions.

The second semester I signed up for Mr. Turner's Shakespeare class again, for graduated students. I became very excited before each class because I knew that at the end of the class I would feel spiritual sublimation, and my pocket would be filled with pearls and diamonds of wisdom. I fulfilled the dream of my beloved Teacher Zhang. I also learned more about the difficulties, complexity, and unpredictability of life, but a pure soul and kind heart would take you far and wide.

An American student who was a little arrogant said to me, "When I saw you come to our class, I thought you were in the wrong classroom, but I didn't expect you to become a class flower!"

"There is nothing difficult in the world," I said, "as long as you are willing to put your heart into it." This Chinese proverb is similar to "Where there is a will there is a way." I firmly believe it and carry it through my whole life. Whatever I want to learn, no matter how difficult it is, I have the confidence and determination to nibble it down.

Let's go back from how I learned Shakespeare in my school years during the cultural revolution. After the order to "resume classes and make a revolution," students came to the classroom every day to study Mao Ze-dong's works in English.

It didn't take long for the news of graduation to arrive. Everyone needed to fill out the allocation form where they wanted to work. From the National Defense Science and Technology Commission to the various industrial ministries, down to the various trading companies in the country.

I never knew what each ministry was for. There were altogether eight industrial ministries. When I found out that the Fourth Electronic Industrial Ministry was engaged in electronics products, I applied to work for it. As soon as the allocation results came out, I was dumbfounded like a thunderbolt on a sunny day. It turned out that the Fourth Electronic Industrial Ministry had many subordinate units in various parts of the country, such as Beijing, Shanghai, Nanjing etc. all big cities. Others were medium size cities such as Wuxi In Jiangsu province, Jingdezhen in Jiangxi province, Baoji in Shaanxi province, Guangyuan in Sichuan province and so on.

I was assigned to Kali in Guizhou province! It was the most remote, the poorest, and the farthest place among all the places. Zhang Guilan, was my classmate and also my good friend and the two of us female students were assigned to Kaili, Guizhou, but we were not together-we were in two different deep ravines on separate jobs. What made me feel most lonely was that she went directly to the factory while I had to go to the artillery farm to do farm work, which was located in a salt flat near Weifang in Shandong province before I went to work in Kali, Guizhou.

I have heard about Guizhou and Shandong but where were the salt flats near Weifang and Kaili? I never heard of them! Maybe they are at the end of the earth? How would I tell my mother and my second elder sister, who was expecting her second child?

With a nervous and an apprehensive heart, I returned home where my mother and my eighth-month-pregnant second elder sister were waiting for me. When I told them the results of the assignment, they couldn't say a word. I was also speechless. The air in the house was so tense and suffocating that it was going to choke people to death.

After a long time, my second elder sister said to me angrily, "Don't go, tell them you are not going there! I'll support you for the rest of your life! " I thanked her in my heart, but how could I let my second elder sister support me for the rest of my life? Since our father passed away, she and her husband had already shouldered the family's financial burden. My mother didn't say a word, but after dinner, when my second elder sister was not present, my mother said to me very seriously, "You can't rely on your sister for a lifetime. Your road still has to be walked by yourself."

My mother's words really surprised me. I didn't know how to interpret them, though the message seemed clear enough. How could she let me go to such a distant place? Didn't she know that my sister loved me the most and really meant what she said? I was puzzled. But subconsciously I felt that my mother's idea was correct.

I chose to go my own way no matter how difficult it was. I had to go to the outside world with my head held high, grit my teeth, and leave home to take the road, even if I did not know where it would lead me. My second elder sister was about to have a baby, so I wrote a letter to the leader in the artillery farm telling them that I had to take some leave because I had to help my mom take care of my older sister. It was approved.

On the evening of September 16, 1968, my second sister started her contractions. There was no taxi then, so I rode a bicycle to Jishuitan Hospital with my second sister sitting on the back rack. We rode through the dark Lake Houhai district. The next morning, my niece Jing-jing was born. I had to board the train going south to Shandong province without waiting for my sister to pass her "Man Yue." (That is a traditional Chinese tradition for the mother to rest for a whole month after she gave birth to a baby). Without saying a word of farewell, I parted with my mother, my sister, and my newborn niece. Our hearts were broken, but there were no tears.

Before leaving Beijing, I went to say goodbye to Hou Yulan, the only junior high school classmate who still had contact with me over the years. Riding a bicycle on the familiar roads in Beijing, Every street was so familiar. I was born and grew up in this city. I remembered what my father once told me: "Our ancestors have been here for more than three hundred years." I said to myself: "Now they don't belong to me, I became an outsider!" Never had I ever imagined that I would be kick out of this beautiful city. Tears burst from my eyes. My heart ached.

It took several times longer than usual to ride to Hou Yulan's home. She didn't go to high school and was already married and had children. As soon as she heard that I was assigned to Kaili, Guizhou and I had to go to the artillery farm in Shandong Province to labor for not knowing how long., she was very sad but helpless. She said decisively: "When you take the bus to Beijing Railway Station, I will ride the tricycle of the shop to bring your luggage to the railway station to meet you." She worked as a saleswoman at Bao Chao Hutong in Gulou East Street. She helped me get on the train to Weifang, Shangdong. She also stuffed a big bag of food for me. (Later, she told me that watching the train leaving, thinking that I had been spoiled since I was a child and now I had to go to the farm alone to work and then I had to go to Guizhou a remote mountain area, she cried and cried). Hou Yulan, where are you now? I do miss you! In order to arrive at Weifang, Shandong during daytime, so I could easily find the artillery farm, I bought a train that left Beijing at night.

When the train was leaving Beijing Railway Station, the radio played the music of "The East is Red" (a song praising Mao). Everyone inside the train stood up and took out the little red book of Chairman Mao's quotations and put it on their chests. My heart was full of anger and helpless sadness, thinking about my older sister who was still in the "month of recovery from delivering my niece." It seemed I also saw the worried and sad eyes of my old mother who always loved and worried about me. I recalled that when I woke up in the middle of the night before I left Beijing, I saw my mother was not in bed, sitting alone in a chair and watching me in a daze. I didn't take out Mao's little red book, but simply let my teardrops run like broken beads falling on the cloth bag sewn by my mother to hold my Yue Qin (Chinese Guitar). This was the first time I left home, left my dear mother, my dear sister, my newborn niece and everyone of my big family and friends. This was the first I had to live on my own, enter the unknown world and puzzled what might happen to me. When the music from the loudspeaker stopped, everyone sat down. I didn't know anyone on the train. I wept for a long time and then fell asleep in a groggy fog. No body looked at me. Nobody cared. I am alone. After I got off the train, following the address on the letter, I found the artillery farm reception place in Wei Fang. The reception staff asked me why I didn't see the reception desk at the train station. I had no idea. I came a month late and there was still a reception desk at the train station?

Nobody told me. They put me on a bus, and after more than two hours, we arrived at the artillery farm on the salt flat in Shouguang County Shandong province.

Chapter 6

Artillery Farm Re-education

It was an endless stretch of salt flats. I saw two rows of red brick houses that were student dormitories. There were a hundred college graduates. We had all been assigned to confidential places throughout the country. Mainly graduates of Qinghua University, Beijing University, Harbin Institute of Military Engineering, Beijing Institute of Light Industry, and other major famous universities. Unlike the college graduates who went to other farms for re-education, we were not reprimanded. Later, I heard that the army leaders in charge of us at our farm were told that these 100 college graduates who had come to receive re-education all had valuable talents, assigned to secret state units, and that we should be treated well.

Many years later, I heard the stories of the hard life of many college and middle school graduates who went up to the mountains, or to the countryside to receive re-education. They were bullied and abused. Many things were unbearable to see or to hear. I think I was lucky to be "re-educated" in a military farm without worrying about not having food or being bullied.

We lived the life of a soldier, getting up at five o'clock every morning to run, sometimes doing some military training, coming back to wash up, eat breakfast, and then going to the fields to do farm work. There was nothing to complain about as far as food was concerned.

We had many varieties and plenty of rice, bread, vegetables and meat dishes every day. Before each meal, we had to line up to sing revolutionary songs and recite Chairman Mao's quotations. We 20 girls slept on wooden planks with top and bottom bunks. Out of 100 college graduates, I was the youngest, 23 years old and the least productive one. When we cleaned the bottom of the canal, almost everyone could carry two buckets of mud with a pole on his or her shoulders. Xi Yinzhu, a graduate of Qinghua University and I, the two of us could not even stand up when we two shared a pole to carry one basket of mud on our shoulder. When I was planting rice, it was simply a torture.

Once a while a frog or some insect appeared in front of my eyes, I was so frightened that I screamed and jumped. Later, I was simply told not to plant rice but just sit on a wooden stool to pluck seedlings. When small animals or bugs appeared, I could lift my feet up with my strong abs and try not to shout for fear of alarming others. Besides, I felt too embarrassed to draw attention to myself and show I was vulnerable or squeamish. The days of laboring in the fields were really painful. I then understood the meaning of helplessness!

At that time, radio stations often announced Chairman Mao's "supreme instructions." As soon as it was broadcast, the whole country had to cheer and celebrate. Therefore, according to the requirements of the artillery regiment headquarters, our student company needed to establish a propaganda team of Mao Ze-dong's thoughts.

Nine people from the 100 college graduates who could play the accordion, huqin (a two-string fiddle), and the harmonica, and those who could sing and dance formed this propaganda team. Of course I was chosen. As soon as there was a holiday, or whenever Mao's instruction was issued, we had to prepare a show for the whole artillery regiment. That was the time I could use all my talents. I wrote lyrics with the tones of folk songs such as Xinjiang, Inner Mongolia, Korean, Tibetan, Han to make new songs, and choreographed movements and dance with these tones. Thus I was given a pleasant nick name, "Art Director."

In order to stage a show on time, the headquarters leader ordered us not to go to the field for labor. Instead, we stayed in the dormitory to practice the singing and dancing, or to rehearse. Most of them didn't have dance training, so I had to teach them. Sometimes I had to change the movements according to everyone's opinion, and then rehearse the programs over and over again. It was a little tiring, but compared to doing farm work in the field, for me, I was in seventh heaven.

Although I was the worst laborer, I tried to work hard to receive re-education. Besides I was simple-minded and was nice to others, so the army commanders and my "classmates" of the student company had a good impression of me and took care of me everywhere. I thank all of them for being so kind to me. No one maliciously teased me or cornered me. It seems God was always protecting me.

I was born in Beiping City (the old name of Peking) and grew up in Beijing (Beiping, Peking and Beijing are the same city). My family had no relatives from the countryside. Coupled with the fact that my parents regarded me as a pearl in the palm of their hands, my world was only to play and to go to school to study. My knowledge out of school was almost zero. For example, what was the difference between horses, donkeys, and mules? I had no idea. What was the difference between rice and weeds? I didn't know. When I saw the sunrise or sunset, the full moon or a crescent moon, I got excited and called everyone to come out to see. Some of them felt strange that I was so nai:ve, "like a kindergartener."

There was no tap water where we lived, but a big tank in front of the dormitory. There was always someone consciously carrying water from a river not far away to fill the tank for everyone to use. I felt that I should carry the water too. I did not expect that carrying water was not only a hard job, but also required a certain amount of skill. I filled the buckets by the river, one in the front and one at the back. I put the pole on my shoulder. It was not easy to stand up against the pain in my right shoulder, but the most awkward dilemma was that I couldn't walk! As soon as I started to walk, the water splashed out of the buckets so high that I got my shoes wet and I couldn't carry them back to the dormitory.

A group of soldiers watched me at a distance and couldn't help laughing. Later, people who were from the countryside taught me the essentials skill of carrying water was to know how to walk. I practiced hard for a week and finally I was able to do it. In fact, mastering the essentials and "rhythm," carrying water was just like dancing. I had to ask my classmates to help me comb my hair and braid my pigtails the next few days, because my right shoulder was red and swollen. I could hardly lift my right arm. However from then on, I could carry two buckets of water with a pole on my shoulder-a piece of cake!

Even though we were treated well at the artillery farm, and ate well, the environment was still very challenging. We had 20 girls sleeping in one room on upper and lower bunk beds. We slept next to each other. Winter came. One time it snowed heavily. Before I got up, I felt someone pouring cold water on my face. Because I was too tired to bother to see what was going on. When the wake-up call whistle rang, I opened my eyes to see two small piles of snow piled up on each side of my ears. It turned out that I was sleeping on the top bunk, and a leaking rooflet the snowflakes drift in from the outside, piling up on each side of my ears. Everyone laughed. I also felt it was funny at that time.

Another experience was terrible. The squad leader moved me from the top bunk to the bottom to sleep. One summer night I slept soundly, and suddenly I felt something moving around my ear. I subconsciously waved my hands and touched a small animal jumping on my chest! I was so scared that I screamed and lifted the mosquito net and immediately drilled into the mosquito net next to me, belonging to my good friend, Guo Sujuan. It turned out to be a rat sneaking into my mosquito net. Everyone was woken up by me and was trying to catch it. I don't remember whether they caught it, but I never dared to go back to my own mosquito net. Guo Sujuan, like a big sister, agreed to my request and let me sleep with her.

Another time, there was a tenth-degree wind. I only heard of such a big wind on the radio. The tiles on the house we lived started to be blown off. A couple of young men climbed up to the roof to fix it. I couldn't remember what I was going to give them. I just remembered when I was about to go back to the dormitory from the corner of the house, suddenly, as if I was kidnapped, the wind pushed me in the opposite direction! I couldn't stop and was forced to run. The terrible thing was that the wind blew me towards a large pigsty dozens of meters away. I wanted to change direction, but I couldn't do anything about it. The girls in our platoon all ran out and stood in front of the house looking at me, laughing. The platoon leader yelled angrily, "You are still laughing! Go and get her back!" The two girls from the Harbin Industry Engineering Institute pulled me back. Otherwise I might have ended up in the pigsty.

It was the first time I was away from home. I couldn't tell you how miserably I suffered from homesickness. Every time I received a letter from my mother, I was sad. One time after dinner, I wanted to read my mother's letter again, but I didn't want people to see me crying, so I walked out. In fact, I was not far from the barracks, about 100 meters.

Holding the letter in my hand, my tears welled out uncontrollably. I simply started to cry. Suddenly I heard a breathing sound behind me. When I looked back, five big dogs surrounded me, staring at me. It scared me to death. I didn't know what to do so I took a step back and they walked a step forward. I wanted to hurry back to the barracks so I turned around and started to run, but they not only ran after me but roared. I ran as fast as possible and fell down in a small puddle of water.

I picked up myself and continued running. The sound of the dogs barking alerted the quartermaster and soldiers, and the students in their rooms. They came out to stop the barking of the dogs. I ran to the door of the girl's dormitory and before entering the room, I leaned against the wall and started to cry loudly. All the girls came out. They didn't know what was happening. I couldn't speak through my tears.

The quartermaster saw that the sleeves of my embroidered cotton jacket were muddy. He asked me if I had been bitten by the dogs. I said no. He said you were crying so hard, I thought you were bitten by a dog! Someone laughed and said, "If you were not bitten by the dogs, then why are you crying? Don't you know that when you see a dog, don't run, the faster you run, the faster they chase you." Later, when I saw a dog, I didn't dare to run away, even if I was afraid. Guo Sujuan, like a big sister, took out a dry cloth from my suitcase and changed it for me. Thank God that when I am in trouble, there will always be someone around me to take care of me. I am so grateful.

Some students did not say it aloud, but they thought that I was too squeamish. Whether that was true or not, the tense life of the farm seemed nothing for others, but it was extremely challenging for me. I disliked the morning exercises- too early; the weather was too cold for me; the mealtime was short, I could not finish my food. Everything was too much for me. I ended up with an infection of my appendicitis. I was sent to the military district's hospital in Zhoucun. The story there is not necessary to tell here.

Two weeks later I was sent back to the farm. No one knew when our re-education would end. I missed my mother so much, and my nephew Xiaochun who grew up with me. With the approval of the army leader, my mother took Xiaochun from Beijing to the farm to see me. I couldn't sleep before their arrival as I was too excited. It had been more than a year since I left home. My 63-year-old mother's hair had all become gray. Cute little Chun was 6 years old. The artillery farm gave us a place to stay. It was only ten minutes' walk from the student company.

We received three meals a day, and I always went to the dining room to bring the food back, and we three enjoyed the temporary pleasure of being together. There had never been an old lady or a child on that large salt flat. My mother was expecting me to leave the farm soon, worrying that I would stay in those desolate salt flats. Thankfully, not long after mom left, we received notice that the re-education was over.

I really wanted to be reassigned or stay somewhere in Shandong. It was much closer to Beijing than Guizhou. I approached the company commander and asked if I could stay in the army. He said, you have important talents cultivated by the state, how can we let you stay? I was very disappointed. The beginning ofJanuary 1970 was the time we left the farm. I was 24 and a half years old. When we were in school, it was forbidden to date. So most of us were single.

Now that we were about to enter society, it is a matter of course to consider dating and marriage. I received several courtship letters, however, either I wasn't interested in having a boyfriend or my biological age and emotional age were not on the same level. I politely declined all the suitors. One of them was a graduate from Beijing University and was assigned to work in Beijing. If I agreed to be his girlfriend, I might be transferred to Beijing. There was also a classmate who had a special affection for me and was willing to accompany me to Guizhou. I Just name a few here. I am deeply grateful to those men who have had affection for me. I respect them, but have never said anything to any other people about them. It remains a beautiful feeling and sweet memories. I cherish their feelings and hide them deeply in my heart.

Chapter 7

Difficult Job Transfer

In Chapter Two you already knew how I met my Prince Charming, and how we became loving husband and wife and had to wait for our reunion in Beijing. This was because the Diplomatic Service Bureau under the Ministry of Foreign Affairs already sent the order for my job transfer to the factory in Kaili, Guizhou where I was working.

Let's go back to 1972 when I was interviewed by the Diplomatic Service Bureau and took the English test. It seemed the transfer should happen next. Can you believe that it took five years for my job transfer?!

After I returned to Kaili, Bing-sheng wrote to me and asked me why the Diplomatic Service had not received my file for such a long time. I was both happy and worried. I went to the Personnel office in my factory and talked to the Director, Wang, who was usually very kind to me. She said, "We are studying it. It will not be fast." Looking at her smiling face, my heart sank. How long do I have to wait? Sadly, in addition to Wang, Bing sheng's anxiety, and my helplessness, there was gossip in the factory, saying that I was not willing to make contributions to build the new factory. The hearsay blamed me in order to transfer back to Beijing, I found an older vice minister-level cadre in Beijing, because they said that only cadres at that level were eligible to transfer their families to Beijing. I really felt greatly insulted, but I could only swallow my anger.

After waiting for a long time, there was still no news. I plucked up enough courage to ask the director of the factory, Mr. Wangqi whether there was a decision on my transfer. I did not expect what this fifteenth-rank cadre said to me, "Your transfer order made the whole factory uneasy. I have received 200 application letters requesting transfers. You have stabbed the honeycomb. What do you want me to do?" His words puzzled me. How could a college graduate in her twenties, newly assigned to the factory, have that much impact?

Many years later, I heard a phrase: envy-jealousy-hate. There are many unexplained attitudes, manifestations, and behaviors in the world. These three words can clearly explain many things. Don't ask why. I think that in the factory where I was located, in addition to the teenage apprentices who went up to the mountains and went to the countryside, most of the technicians, master workers, including administrative leaders, were sent to that ravine from the Beijing Factory under an order. I now understand too well the psychology of people at that time. Nobody wanted to leave Beijing but due to political pressure, one had to behave actively, and answer the call to go to the deep mountains. How could others not be jealous of my returning to Beijing?

It lasted for quite a while, and then I went to find the military representative, Lao Li, who came from the Third Department of the General Staff, dispatched to our factory. Lao Li was the number one leader of the factory party committee. I told him about my situation. He said, "Now our country needs foreign language talents like you, but I can't make the decision alone, so let me hold a party committee meeting as soon as possible to discuss your transfer." Later, I heard that when the party committee discussed my transfer issue, there were a total of five people. The three military deputies all agreed to my transfer, but Director Wang Qi of the factory and Chief Engineer Ni did not agree to let me go. By a show of hands, 3 to 2, my work transfer was approved in accordance with the stipulation within the Party that the minority obey the majority.

I really didn't understand, was I that important? In a factory with thousands of people, I was simply a small potato. Deputy Wang Jun, who was one of the five party committee members in charge of personnel business, informed the personnel office that my transfer had been approved. However, the chief of the personnel office, Ms. Wang, said that she could not send my personal file to Beijing . She needed to report it to the headquarters 083 for approval. Wait, wait, wait. At this time, the news came that the military representatives were leaving and returning to Beijing.

I suddenly felt that the situation was not in my favor. If they were all gone, who could speak for me? On the day that Yang Jihou, a military representative, left the factory, I chased him to the location of 083 in Duyun. I found the personnel office one level higher than my factory. The person who received me was Xiao Zhang, who used to work in my friend Zhang Guilan's factory. When I asked about my transfer, she told me that the report from my factory did not mention that Beijing needed you to work in the foreign diplomatic circle, but simply wrote a sentence, "She has a boyfriend in Beijing and asked for a transfer. The factory approved her request."

God, how ridiculous this was! After I listened to it, I had the heart to kill them. They didn't tell the whole story. Xiao Zhang also said, "We have to report to the National Defense Industrial Office in Guiyang for approval. However, your case will certainly not be approved. Your boyfriend can't be counted as a family relationship. You have to ask your factory personnel office to resend the letter explaining that the reason for your transfer is the need to work in the foreign diplomatic circle." I had no time to get angry and immediately found Lao Yang, who had not yet left. He was also one of the three people who agreed to my transfer in the meeting of the factory party committee. I told him about the situation. He said with a bitter smile, "I didn't expect them play tricks with words on the paperwork."

I asked him if he could go to the 083 Personnel Office to explain the real situation. He is a cadre of the army, and a representative of our factory. Definitely he would be more convincing than anything I said. He did go to tell the truth. Then, Xiao Zhang said that we still had to report to the upper level, the National Defense Industrial Office in Guiyang. You'd better ask your factory to re-submit a document as soon as possible to explain the reason for your transfer.

I went back to the factory to find the chief of the personnel office, Ms. Wang, who now didn't even have a fake smile. Very impatiently she said, "Okay." I obviously felt that as soon as the military deputies left, the cadres of this factory would collude to prevent me from going back to work in Beijing.. But people under the eaves of others had to bow their heads. I couldn't do anything about it. Patiently, I waited, waited, and waited. There was nothing from the National Defense Industrial Office about my transfer. I took advantage of a business trip to Guiyang and found the office of the National Defense Industrial Office.

It was a Saturday. It was already noon after my meeting. I only had half a day to inquire about my transfer. I did not dare to delay the time for lunch in order to find the location of the National Defense Industry Office. I was so hungry that I could hardly walk. I needed to find a restaurant to eat and then keep going. But there was no dish in the restaurant that was not spicy. Guizhou people eat spicy food no less than Sichuan people. The dish had no oil, dry and spicy. I hadn't learned to eat spicy food yet. I found a little booth on the street and I bought a dry apple and a pear that was not yet the size of an egg. There was no where I could sit so I sat on the side of the road and nibbled on the apple and pear. Although unlike a beggar, the scene of an over twenty years old girl sitting on the side of the road in Guiyang and nibbling on fruit, must have been very funny. It should be miserable but I get rid of that unhealthy feeling. The perseverance spirit of a Manchu girl helped me to have my head on. I had not time to pity myself. I need to fight for the future of my life. However, I will never forget that scene!

It was more than three o'clock in the afternoon when I found the Defense Industrial Office. The compound was quiet. I hope they hadn't left their office. I was looking for someone to ask where the personnel office was. There was a young girl on the other side of the road who spoke to me, "Master Li, how come you are here?" As soon as she asked me, I was so happy that I was going to jump!

It turned out that she was Xiao Liu who used to work in the workshop of my factory. When I was the secretary of the Youth League, I had to persuade those who disagreed to accept her to join the Youth League. Because when she was nineteen years old as an apprentice, she fell in love with a military officer. She did well in every aspect. As the leader of the youth league, I said she was serious about her work, gentle, caring for the group. Now she was 19 years old, just entering her adulthood. We had no reason to disapprove her to joining the Youth League. Later she got married and was transferred to Guiyang where her husband worked.

I didn't expect to meet her in a situation like this. I briefly explained what I was going to ask the personnel office about my job transfer. She said that her husband was working in that compound. She could ask him to go to the personnel office to help me find out about the status of my job transfer. After waiting less than an hour, the answer came back: The Personnel Office of the National Defense Industrial Office did not receive an explanation from our factory that I was transferred to Beijing mainly due to the need of work, but only that I had a boyfriend in Beijing. Nothing had changed! The Commissioner also said that a boyfriend was not legally considered a family member. How come the factory and 083 approved her transfer? Yet they were about to issue a document not approving my transfer!

After I heard the story, I was very disappointed, but did not feel that this was the end of the world. After all, I prevented them from sending the documents of non-approval to the factory, so that the decision of the original party committee that I could transfer would not be overturned! It's dangerous! How "clever" their means were. Since God let me make acquaintances at a critical time, and know the truth, there is salvation. I begged them not to send the non-approved documents to the factory. They asked me to contact Beijing again. The person in the office said that Beijing could send the transfer order directly to the Defense Industrial Office. I said that I would ask Wang Bingsheng to explain the situation to the Personnel Office of the Beijing Diplomatic Service Bureau under the Ministry of Foreign Affairs to send a letter of transfer order directly to the National Defense Industrial Office. He said let's wait.

I did not know whether to be happy or angry, whether I should laugh or cry. At least I felt that I put out a burning fire. I did not come to Guiyang in vain. Xiao Liu was my savoir that day. Later, I learned some famous sayings, "To love others is to love yourself," and "Good people are rewarded." This has been proved countless times in my life. Many times when I was in danger, there was always an invisible hand holding me, and helping me escape the danger. I was very thankful for Xiao liu and her husband. With a heart full of sorrow and anger, I returned to my factory in Kali. After spending a sleepless night, I went to Mr. Wang Yi, the deputy director of the factory, to file a complaint and also vent my grievances and the despair that I had suppressed for so long in my heart.

He wasn't in his office. The secretary told me he was holding a meeting in the conference room with the section directors. I knew that it would take the whole morning, and I really didn't want to wait, so I went to the conference room, saying loudly through the window, "Comrade Wang Yi, please come out!"

Mr. Wang Yi was not from the old factory in Beijing He was transferred from the Ministry of Agriculture to the third-line factory. Because his office and radio room were in the same hall, we usually bumped into each other often. He appreciated my working style and said that I was very serious in handling any matter. Now he saw me full of anger.

He said kindly, "What's the matter, Xiao Li, I'm in a meeting."

I said, " I just came back from Guiyang and this couldn't wait. Why didn't Zhong Shilin (a clerk in the personnel office) didn't say that I was needed for foreign affairs work in the report of my transfer, but only wrote about my boyfriend?" I spoke so loudly and the windows were open that the directors inside were listening to our conversation and were silent. Mr. Wang Yi pulled me aside and whispered, "You can't do anything this way.

I'll ask the Personnel Office later." He added another sentence that stunned me, "After all, you still have hope to go back to Beijing. We're going to have to stay here forever!" Looking at his helpless expression, I was dumbfounded. My job transfer seemed to have so many obstacles. I was extremely depressed.

Then the political situation got worse. With the approval of

Mao Zedong, the CPC Central Committee launched a political campaign criticizing Lin Biao (a general who was supposed to be Mao's successor but was shot down on his way to escape China) and Confucius (They were aiming Premier Zhou Enlai). My transfer was suspended again. Discouragement and disappointment were my mood at the time. In 1976, there were many major events happening in China: The three Chinese leaders Premier Zhou Enlai, Marshal Zhu De, and Chairman Mao Ze-dong died within months of one another. In the same year, on July 28, a 7.8 magnitude earthquake occurred in Tangshan, 104 miles from Beijing. The whole city was destroyed. I had no mind to work at all, so I took a leave of absence to return to Beijing in August.

Living in a tent shelter in the courtyard with Bingsheng, "enjoying" the aftershocks, and sharing hardships with relatives were much better than being alone in Guizhou. On October 6 of 1976, Hua Guofeng, the acting premier and minister of public security of the State Council, Ye Jianying, vice chairman and secretary general of the Central Military Commission, Li Xian nian, vice premier of the State Council, and others, with the support of Wang Dongxing, leader of the Central Guard Force and director of the General Office of the CPC Central Committee, carried out an arrest operation and detained the Gang of Four, Jiang Qing(Mao's wife), Zhang Chunqiao, Yao Wen-yuan, and Wang Hongwen, who had been accused of harming the country and the people.

I was 31 years old. The idea of having a child finally began to kick in. I returned to Kaili, Guizhou pregnant. Three months or so, an unfortunate thing happened in my factory. Bi Xiaowu, who was the sister of my good friend Bi Lianrong, had bone cancer and passed away. Xiaowu was beautiful and a good basket player. She was only 15 years old! I was so sad that I didn't want to talk to anyone. I wanted to be left alone. So I carried an 8 pound thermos bottle of hot water to my office on the fifth floor (there was no elevator). I wanted to drink some hot water in my own office and calm down my disturbed and sad heart. I knew her classmates were making wreaths and preparing for the next day's funeral service. Thinking that her young life was lost so quickly, worrying about how her parents, brothers and sisters could bear it, I really felt down and miserable. Looking at the pile of hard coals by the stove, I simply sat on a small stool to start to smash the coal blocks with a hammer because the next day I needed smaller pieces of coal for the stove.

According to state regulations, Guizhou belongs to the south region and no heating system was provided, but the winter in Guizhou was cold and wet, so each office was equipped with a coal-burning stove as a heater. After smashing the coal for quite a while, I listlessly went back to my dorm.

I suddenly felt a little cold under my lower body, A little red at first glance, I didn't know what to do, I went to Master Tao's house, and as soon as she heard about it, she immediately said, no, you have to go to the hospital quickly. Her husband, Lao Zhao, was the chief of the security office. He immediately drove the firetruck (there was no ambulance at that time) and took me to Kaili's 818 Hospital.

The doctor checked me and said I should be hospitalized to protect the fetus. After I was arranged in an empty ward, they all left, leaving me alone. It was dark outside. I was so sad that I couldn't hold back the tears that had been accumulating for the whole day. I cried when I lay under the quilt. After a while, the doctor came. She comforted me and said, "Please don't be sad. I will do my best to help you keep the child."

After staying in the hospital for a few days, there was no movement of the fetus. Several experiments were done. Then the doctor said disappointedly, she could not hear the fetus' heartbeat. After Bingsheng learned my situation, he really worried about me. He called and said that he couldn't leave his work and the whole family decided to send his younger sister to Guizhou to take care of me.

Several of my best friends came to the hospital to help me to decide what to do. Master Tao asked the doctor if it would be dangerous if I took the train back to Beijing immediately. The reply was that she was an elderly mother-to be and it was estimated that there would be no miscarriage on the road if the doctor gave me a shot. Everyone asked for my opinion. I said, "I am Going back to Beijing!" That evening, Master Tao and Master Liu put me on a train to Beijing (Kaili already had a direct train to Beijing). I risked miscarriage on the trip, bravely took the train for two nights and three days, and finally returned to Bingsheng. My heart calmed down at last. It looked like a crooked seedling found a big tree for support.

In many situations where there might be danger (I have always been in danger since I was born), I was always saved. God, I am grateful! The next day we went to Beijing Maternity Hospital for examination. The doctor said that she could not hear any movement and she would do another experiment test the next day. On the night I got home, I thought, there was Bingsheng, and there was a doctor. I was not afraid of anything. I started to sing folk songs happily, such as "North Wind Blow" "Embroidering Gold Plaque." Suddenly my lower part started to bleed. Bingsheng immediately called a car and sent me to the maternity hospital. Before the doctor came, I could not control myself, and blood spread all over the place. We could not find anything to clean things up and I felt so embarrassed. The nurse pushed me into the ward. The doctor immediately performed an abortion surgery.

Later, I saw those scenes on movies. Stories of maternal bleeding happened. For example, Hu Niu in "Camel Shoko", played by Si Qin Gao Wa; The daughter-in-law in Alive played by Gong Li. They all died of maternal bleeding when they were delivering babies. I was so lucky. But who could guarantee that I wouldn't be the unfortunate woman? I immediately wrote a letter to the factory and asked for a month's leave. We lost our first child. Neither of us was sad, but my mother-in-law regretted this. However, she cooked very nutritious food for me, and I rested for a month.

I remembered returning to the Guizhou factory at the end of March. Three months later, when Deng Xiaoping resumed his work, on July 15th, 1977, Our factory received another transfer letter from the Ministry of Foreign Affairs. When I asked Mr. Yang, the new section chief of the Personnel Office to sign it, he said that he should report to 083 again to approve it. I said, "Chief Yang, my job transfer has been delayed for five years, please simply let me go." His son, Yang Tiezheng, used to work with me at the factory radio station and we were on good terms. Chief Yang said, all right. He signed the transfer letter and also agreed not to report to 083 for approval. He let me go.

My heart was full of blossoming flowers, but I didn't dare to delay any longer. As the saying goes, "When night is long, any dream might happen." I decided to leave Kali right away to go back to Beijing. I told a few good friends of mine that I would not take anything with me, and divide my belongings among themselves. On July 17, 1977, I took a few clothes in a small bag and left the ravine that had locked me in for eight years. On the train for three days I was so excited that I couldn't close my eyes. It was like a dream. The torturing experience of being trapped in that deep and remote mountain gave me nightmares for many years even after I returned to Beijing. I often woke up crying . In my dreams, my hair turned grey because my hopeless waiting and waiting to be transferred back to Beijing. When I woke up, I was so glad that it was just a dream, but tears were still in my eyes. The belief that "persistence was the key to success" became stronger and stronger in my mind.

Two months later, my good friends sent back my belongings, including the hardwood, Phoebe, I bought from local farmers. After several years of tribulation, torture, pain, and disappointment, I finally returned to Bingsheng, my husband, and my mom and siblings, people I missed day and night.

Why did I write about this transfer in such a detail? Because this job transfer took 5 years! It was the most troublesome thing, the most helpless and the most painful happening in my life. It had separated me and my dear husband for all that time, tormented me for several years, and wasted my youth. It also brought me and my family pain that was difficult to express in words. The unexpected behavior of people, and the complexity of the world gave me an unforgettable lesson for a lifetime. Writing in such detail is also a nostalgia for me and my first love, remembering my first husband Wang Bingsheng and our years of suffering together. He had been faithfully and patiently waiting for me, caring for me, inspiring me. In 1975, he also escorted me to my factory in Kaili, Guizhou, where he cooked for me every day. He is a big tree that will always stand in my heart.

Speaking of that job transfer, I would like to tell a story that touched me very much. On February 21, 1972, a major event occurred that shocked the whole world: US President Nixon arrived in Beijing to visit China before the two countries established formal diplomatic relationship since new China was founded in 1949. I happened to be back in Beijing to visit my mother. On that day, with great curiosity, I went to Tiananmen Square and stood in front of the Forbidden City with thousands of Chinese, waiting for Nixon's motorcade to pass through. The weather was cloudy. The crowd was quiet. "Here they come." Someone whispered. Soon a long convoy came from the east of Chang'an Street. After the police cars drove by, a luxury car with two national flags, a Chinese flag and an American flag, came closer and closer. I suppose Nixon must have been sitting inside. Unfortunately the curtains in the car were not lifted. As soon as the convoy passed, people quietly dispersed. I didn't know other people's thoughts, but my heart was very excited: the isolation between China and the United States was coming to an end. The process of normalization of relations began. Those of us who study English should be very useful!

Sure enough, later, I heard Premier Zhou Enlai asked,

"Where have all the interpreters we trained gone?" Culture Revolution broke out in 1966 and no universities enrolled any students since then until 1977. When we graduated in 1968, most of the students of foreign language colleges and universities were assigned to farms, or to various parts of the country (Actually there were very few universities with foreign language studies in the whole country. Beijing Foreign Language College, Beijing Foreign Trade Institute, and Beijing Foreign Affairs University were the biggest.) As a result, both the Ministry of Foreign Affairs and the Ministry of Foreign Trade were looking for graduates from their affiliated colleges. A condition to go back to Beijing to work as interpreters was that they could not start a family in the local area, except if both husband and wife were graduates of foreign language colleges and they still maintained a certain level of foreign language skill. I was so far away in Guizhou and didn't know all this.

An old classmate of mine saw that my aging mother was alone in Beijing. Although there was a son and daughter-in-law around her, mother and daughter-in-law did not get along. They did not even talk to each other. This classmate of mine went to the Ministry of Foreign Trade to find Mr. Miao Junqing who was in charge of recalling the former students to come back to Beijing to work. My old classmate mentioned the difficulties of my family and asked Mr. Miao for help. He also "lied" to say that I was his girlfriend. As a matter of fact, he was already in the list of recalled students. Later, I learned that only one of the two of us could return to Beijing. Then he changed his word to tell Mr. Miao that we were not boyfriend and girlfriend. My family situation needed me to go back to Beijing to take care of my aging mother. I didn't know whether Mr. Miao Junqing knew me and knew the situation of my family, or sympathized with the situation, he did send the job transfer order of the Ministry of Foreign Trade to my factory in Kaili, Guizhou. I didn't know anything about these situations until much later.

Only when I went to the personnel office of my factory toinquire about my job transfer to the Ministry of Foreign Affairs,

I heard Chief Wang said, "Don't ask anymore. We haven't finished handling the job transfer request from Foreign Ministry's Affairs and now the Ministry of Foreign Trade's job transfer order has also come. We don't know how to answer it yet!" Maybe they never answered the Ministry of Foreign Trade at all. No wonder a few years later, I heard that Mr. Miao had misunderstood me: saying that I only wanted to go to the Ministry of Foreign Affairs and could care less of the offer from the Ministry of Foreign Trade. Oh my God, I'm a graduate of the Foreign Trade Institute. There were a lot of classmates and schoolmates working there, how could I choose not to back to the Ministry of Foreign Trade? This misunderstanding was impossible and there was no need to explain.

That classmate who went to Mr. Miao twice to help me transfer back to Beijing missed the opportunity. It was delayed for several years before he was transferred back to the Ministry of Foreign Trade. I heard all these stories later. However, I've been grateful to him for the rest of my life. Sometimes I think that the relationships between people are incredible and beyond explanation. I deeply appreciated his selfless help.

I feel that I am really a lucky woman in this world. All these gentlemen who love me selflessly, persistently, deeply, fully support me and wish me to live a better life, are so worthy of my writing. They are an integral part of my life. I learned a great deal from them. They are all gods and heroes in my heart. No matter what other people think of me, whether they criticize me, or despise me, I could care less. I know in my heart that the world, the bizarre, the inconceivable arrangement of fate and life are beyond our control. These nice people will always stand tall in my heart and deserve my lifelong gratitude, respect and love!

Chapter 8

Ten Years of Life in Beijing

In July 17, 1977, I came back to Beijing, my hometown, back to my mother, my siblings and my dear husband, Bingsheng, starting my long dreamed life.

When we were in college, we were told that our future job would be intermediate or advanced interpreters and translators. Although it had been several years since I left the institute, thanks to the English materials sent to me by my friend Wang Shumian, I practiced speaking and listening English secretly at nights, plus Bingsheng and I had been communicating and speaking in English. So my English was not forgotten.

The first day when I went to work at Tanzanian Embassy stationed in Beijing, there was no language barrier. The Tanzanian ambassador to China, Mr. and Mrs. Lucinda and other diplomats were very satisfied with my work. In addition to translation work, I also handle visas to Tanzania. I would accompany the Ambassador, the Ambassador's wife and all the diplomats and their ladies on their errands. During my five years working at the Tanzanian Embassy, 13 children were born in Beijing. Our daughter Wang Xiao-nan was born on April 26, 1978. We named her Xiao-nan (also known as Nannan and Nancy) . The pronunciation of xiao means to know. Nan has several meanings: 1. The south; 2. Hardship and difficulties; 3. A hard wood tree called Phoebe, sturdy and strong, high quality for anything. Bing sheng and I named our daughter Xiaogan which means to know her mother's difficulties in Guizhou, in the southern part of China. We also hope that she would become as strong and valuable as the tree, Phoebe. She lived up to our expectations. We also gave her an English name: Nancy. Nancy's nickname in our neighborhood was Little Princess Wang because of her special walking demeanor and unexpected reserved manner. To raise Nancy was our most happy experiences.

When I was five months pregnant, my mother had a cerebral thrombosis. Bingsheng received a call from my sister about my mother. He worried about me, so he told me that he had to accompany foreign guests to the Great Wall and come back late. At the end of the day, I felt unsettled. Before I left work, I called his colleagues at the Canadian Embassy stationed in Beijing where he worked. I asked when Bingsheng would return. The colleague inadvertently said that he had gone to visit my mother who was being taken to the hospital. It was a shock. I was anxious about my mother and I was sad that Bingsheng had to tell a white lie. He was afraid that I was five months pregnant and might worry too much about my mother, and that I would be too emotional. A high respect arose for him that he alone would carry the burden of taking care of two people at the same time. I was really grateful that I had such a caring husband.

My mother's life was saved but she couldn't live by herself anymore. She couldn't even speak or walk. My eldest sister lived in Tianjin. My second elder sister lived in Ningxia. My younger sister lived in Huairou, the suburb of Beijing. Even though my older brother and his family were in Beijing and shared the same house with my mother, but his wife and my mother had not spoken to each other for years. Bingsheng was obligated to take my mother to our home.

Watching him carry my mother upstairs, my eyes were full of tears. In addition to his busy work, he had to take care of me and my mother every day, purchasing groceries, cooking, and washing. I had never seen him frown or complain. Where in the world can one find such a good husband, a good son-in-law! Over the years, the Li family has held high esteem for him.

Here I also want to write the story of Nancy's birth, which was a drama, a comedy, and a burlesque.

On April 25, 1978, at 1:30 p.m., I had just finished eating lunch with my mother and suddenly my stomach began to hurt. I knew that my due date had passed a few days already and I had read some books about fertility. I knew I should go to the hospital. I immediately prepared a little package and made a piece of dough. I told my mother that I was going to the hospital for a physical examination and asked her to tell Bingsheng to make some steamed buns after his work. I rode my bicycle towards Beijing Maternity Hospital in Nanchizi Hutong. Yes, I went to the hospital on my own bike. Taking a pregnant woman to the hospital on a bicycle seemed to be a "template" in my life.

On September 15,1968, my second elder sister was going to give birth to her daughter; it was I who rode bicycle to take her to Jishuitan Hospital passing by Lake Houhai in dark. On January 22, 1970, my second elder sister was going to give birth to a son. I carried her on my bike passing by the cold Lake Houhai to Jishuitan Hospital to deliver her son.

This time it was my turn to deliver my own daughter. It seemed I was well-prepared. In the kingdom of bicycle, I was like a bird flying everywhere easily. Later when I returned to Beijing around the age of 70, I could still ride freely on the crowded roads of Beijing. From my home to Beijing Maternity Hospital, it took more than 40 minutes to ride the bike. I knew that the first baby would not be born immediately. It took a long time for the uterus to open- if it was fast it took a few hours; if it is slow it might take three days. Anyway, it is different from a woman to another. Not a pleasant experience. In old Chinese saying, "To deliver a baby, the mother has passed a door of death".

Bingsheng was so worried about me that every time when we went to the store he put his hand around me in order not to let other people bump into me. I couldn't let him worry and more importantly, my old mother who just had a cerebral thrombosis needed him to be around, so I didn't call him. A book described that uterine pain began in about half an hour at the beginning and then intervals gradually shortened between the pains. I felt the pain two times on the road to the hospital. Each time when I felt the pain, I stopped the bicycle with my right foot next to the curb and waited until the pain passed. Then I continued to ride the bike. In less than an hour I arrived at the maternity hospital. I parked my bike and went to the office. The nurse asked me where my husband was. I said he was busy at work and had to take care of my sick mother after work, so I came by bicycle myself. She said very suspiciously, how do you know that you are going to give birth, is it near the due date, I don't know if you can be admitted to the hospital, etc.

At that time, the Cultural Revolution had just ended. I didn't know why the doctors and nurses all talked very rudely like a machine gun. I had experienced so many unfair things in the world. I was used to the rude behavior. I didn't care about their attitude. After a while the doctor came and after the examination, she said, accept her to the hospital. I had to call Bingsheng to take home my bike when he had time because my bike was still parked outside the hospital. He hurried to the hospital and wanted to see me, but they wouldn't let him in. He had to go home worried and disappointed.

From 10 o'clock on that night, I was in excruciating pain. My back and stomach hurt really bad. There was no comfort words and nobody came to see me. On the contrary, they always came to "attack" and "lecture" me together. When it hurt, I pulled the leg of the tablet to vent my pain. I didn't want to shout like other pregnant women, how embarrassing! I always wanted to go to the toilet as if the pain was better when I walked. After going two or three times, the nurse got angry at me and said loudly, "Why don't you bear it? What if you give birth to the child in the toilet?" About midnight, the doctor put me to the delivery bed. I could hardly move. I was hungry, tired and in pain. I really felt that it was better to die than to suffer. Who would have known it would be so hard and painful to deliver a baby? I'm never going to have a second child again. The time of contractions was getting shorter and shorter. In the same delivery room there were four of us pregnant women, the other three left one after another after giving birth to their children. Then two more came in, also left after delivering their babies. I was still lying there alone and the nurses and doctors were very anxious. Now that I am writing this, I really don't know whether I should laugh or cry because a dramatic oral war of words began. The protagonists were me and the doctors and nurses in the obstetrics department of Beijing Maternity Hospital.

I heard a woman saying, "This one has been lying here for a long time while everyone else has gone, including the ones who came in later than her." Another said: "Her condition, the shape and size of her pelvis, were perfect for having children, how can she not work hard?" I couldn't help it, so I interjected, "You said I'm not trying hard? I don't have any strength at all." There came another one who said even more harshly, "If you don't know how to deliver a baby then you shouldn't get pregnant!" I thought it was too much so I retorted, "This child was not in my plans. It was accidentally conceived." She got irritated and said, "You see she has all the strength to argue with us, but no energy to deliver a baby! I have never seen it."

The nurses' duty should be to sympathize with the patient and to help the patient relieve their pain. They should be angels in white, but when I needed the most care and help, I heard such harsh things, in a reprimanding tone. China was known as a country of etiquette, and people should care for and help each other, especially when a new mother of 33 gave birth to her first child, but all I heard were reprimands, ridicule, and attacks. How ridiculous and how vicious! Actually, I should not blame them for being so unreasonable and rude. The Cultural Revolution washed away people's nature of kindness as if the fiercer they spoke, the more heroic they were.

Benevolent, kind, courteous, frugal and gentle, these fine qualities are written in The Analects and are part of the culture of Chinese society, but these fine traditions were criticized and castrated during the Cultural Revolution. To be mean and rude were considered normal behavior. There was nothing I could do. I had been out of the house since 1:30 p.m., not a sip of water or a bite of food were given to me. I was so exhausted, and I didn't want to hear them scold me anymore, so I simply closed my eyes and said nothing. However, I heard some nurse saying, "Hey, look, now she went to sleep!" She also shouted at me loudly, "Don't you go to sleep! Do you want your child or not?"

I replied in a nonchalant voice, "Of course I want my child!" By this time, it was already dawn, about half past six in the morning. The doctors and nurses began to change shifts. I heard the voice of a new doctor. She said, "You have been lying here all night. Now we will help you, but we need you to work hard to give birth to the child; otherwise, it will be dangerous to the child." I said OKAY. The contractions came again, and everyone was shouting together: "Try hard! Push hard!" I exerted my greatest strength and I heard the doctor say that I had to be cut open with a pair of scissors. I said whatever you do, I don't care now. It was over 7 o'clock in the morning when my daughter came to this world! At first, I had no feelings for her. She tortured me for more than 16 hours. I was not prepared to be a mother. Looking at her plump little round face, I thought to myself, "Is this my daughter? Have I become a mother?"

What a blissful thing to be in love, to get married, to conceive and to have children. Yet all happiness is accompanied by pain. It can send you to heaven or send you to hell; You can be flattered and enjoy the pleasures of the world, or you may be lost and tortured. That's life! It is undeniable that I was originally a simple girl who sometimes did not quite live up to a standard of an adult, or unbelievably na"ive, but after going through all layers of "pollution" and "corrosion" in my life, I was forced to change.

Nancy's growth was very smooth. She has a big forehead, curly hair, chubby little hands and feet, never crying, she drew attention and loving eyes everywhere I took her. Bingsheng and I worked during the day and I came home at noon to breastfeed her. We hired a nanny to take care of my mother and Nancy. My family was full of joy.

Unfortunately, my mother left us at the age of 73, a month after Nancy turned one year old. As the saying goes, 73, or 84 is the threshold year for seniors. My mother saw my daughter, but my daughter could not remember her grandmother. I am now a grandmother. I have allowed my grandchildren enjoy all the love I can give to them. Nancy has a grandfather, grandmother, aunts, uncles, cousin sisters, and cousin brothers. The third generation of our Li family has a total of 12 third generations, and Nancy is the youngest. There are 6 cousins from Wang Bing-sheng's family. Nancy has a total of 17 cousins. Every weekend, Bing sheng and I either went back to his parents' house or entertained guests at our own home. To this day, these cousins still interact with each other. Nancy is popular everywhere. She is a lucky one. I never told her that when she was born, her mother rode a bike to maternity hospital and suffered a lot, nor did I tell her how the doctors and nurses counted me down and how we fought orally. I wrote it here in such detail; it was for her. One day when she reads my autobiography, she will compare how lucky and happy she was in the United States from pregnancy to deliver her two children.

In the blink of an eye, five years went by in my work at the Tanzanian Embassy in Beijing. After the formal establishment of diplomatic relations between the United States and China on January 1, 1979, the U.S. Commercial Office was also established in 1982. After being interviewed by the first U.S. Commercial Counsellor, Mr. Melvin Searls asked me to work for the U.S. Commercial Section (at that time, the U.S. Embassy set up The Commercial Section in Jianguo Hotel). The five years I worked in The Commercial Section was also five years allowing me to give my full potentials and abilities. I had helped countless American companies, politicians, and entrepreneurs understand China, get acquainted with their Chinese counterparts and politicians. I have also helped various Chinese commercial departments and companies, including units and enterprises in Shenyang, Wuhan, Lanzhou, and other places, to make contact with the American business community.

I also cooperated with the U.S. Embassy to receive countless national, large and small business delegations, negotiating delegations, often unprepared to be called to do on-site interpreting. When President Reagan visited China, the seats at the returning banquet were all arranged by me. When Mr. Randt , the first secretary of The Commercial Section at that time (who later became the

U.S. ambassador to China) wrote me a letter of recommendation when I applied to further study in the U.S., he said that the person any American businessman needed to meet when he came to The Commercial Section was actually Ms. Li because she knew the situation in China very well and the phone numbers of all the Chinese units were in her head.

Because the officers of the Commerce Section were very satisfied with my work, they arranged to send me to the United States to "study" as a reward, but they did not reach an agreement with the Foreign Diplomatic Service Bureau, so Mr. Searls arranged my "study" at the American Commercial Section stationed in Hong Kong for a few days as an award. In short, my work, family, and life were very ideal.

Bingsheng also did a good job at the Canadian Embassy stationed in China. When the United Nations recruited the first group of simultaneous interpreters in China, Bing-sheng signed up for the exam. Among hundreds of people across the country, he stood out as one of the last 30 candidates. This time he missed the opportunity to go abroad again. Instead of being discouraged, he said happily, "If they really want me to go, I feel reluctant, because I don't want to leave you and Nancy behind." We also moved from the guest house into the service bureau dormitory building in the Embassy district and had our own peaceful residence, a beautiful home: no noise of public transportation, and a very quiet and nice environment. We both had subsidies for working in the Embassies. It was really a happy little family.

Many people have asked me, why did you leave that nice workplace, your ideal husband, and lovely daughter to come to the United States alone? I've asked myself this question countless times, too. Being governed by the Chinese system and embarrassing situations at work are the main reasons. That I am an easily unsatisfied person is another reason. Let me give a few examples of how I was embarrassed at work. Those were part of the reasons why I decided to leave my position and came to the U.S.

In the unit where I worked at that time, I couldn't say or do many things that I did not understand. That really got on my nerves. For example, When Bingsheng and I got married, he was working at the Kuwaiti Embassy stationed in China. The ambassador had great respect for him. However, the Chinese leader asked him to take three days off, saying that he needed to be hospitalized for an examination and could not tell the ambassador that he was getting married. Why? They said it might bring too much trouble. What logic was that? Marriage is a big thing in one's life and using hospitalization as an excuse for taking leave of absence seemed so strange. Was there a curse on him? Another example: When I gave birth to my daughter, the wife of the ambassador, Mrs. Lusinda of the Tanzanian Embassy stationed in China where I worked at the time, wanted to come to the hospital to visit me. The leader asked another interpreter to tell the ambassador's wife that Xiao Li would not agree to her visit because it was not very convenient. Such an answer made the ambassador's wife very unhappy.

There was another situation that bothered me very much. The Diplomatic Service Bureau, where we work is a bureau under the Ministry of Foreign Affairs of China. There is an unwritten rule that after ten years of working there, you will be sent to be a diplomat. I heard that the Chinese ambassador to Australia needed a young couple who could speak English and someone recommended Bing-sheng and I to work for him. Being a diplomat was an honorable position for us who were foreign language students. However, the Personnel Office of the Service Bureau did not let us go. The answer was that Wang

Bing-sheng and his wife could not leave their positions because one was the pillar of the Canadian Embassy in China, and the other was the pillar of the Commercial Section of the U S Embassy in China.

It was not a bad thing to really value us like this, but the ranking work that followed later on upset me. After we graduated, we did not have a rank or title. The interpreter and translator job we were assigned in foreign embassies in China were uniformly called Chinese Secretaries. Now it was the first time to evaluate our work and assigned the rank of section chief, deputy section chief, and section member. It was also stated that the rating is not tied to wages. When discussing the rank of Bingsheng and I, a leader said that this couple could not be ranked the same. Only one was section chief and the other had to be deputy section chief; otherwise the impact would not be good. Weren't the achievements of work taken into consideration? What about the saying of the pillars at work? It may be that I valued the ranking too much. I could not get myself free of desire for fame and fortune. Anyway, it bothered and disappointed me for a long time. Later in my old age, I became realized that everything is empty. From learning "Heart Sutra" I understand that:

Form is no other than emptiness, Emptiness no other than form. Form is only emptiness, Emptiness only form. Feeling, thought, and choice, consciousnessitself, are the same as this.

All things are by nature void. They are not born or destroyed, nor are they stained or pure. Nor do they wax or wane.

So in emptiness, noform,

No feeling, thought, or choice, Nor is there consciousness. No eye, ear, nose, tongue, body, mind;

No colour, sound, smell, taste, touch, or what the mind takes hold of, nor even act of sensing.

I hope I learned these concepts.

Another thing happened that made me feel like swallowing a fly. I couldn't spit it out even if I felt nauseous. As soon as the Commercial Section of the U.S. Embassy in China was established, I was selected by the first U.S. Commercial Counsellor, Mr. Melvin Sears, to work there. Five years later, the Commercial Section expanded: from just two officials and me to five officials, two secretaries, two Chinese drivers, and three Chinese employees. All five officials were fluent in Chinese. My main task seemed only to arrange lunches and banquets and seating positions. I was a little bored.

Then the chief interpreter of the Culture Section of the U.S. Embassy, Mr. Wang Tuoqiang, told me he would be sent abroad to work as a diplomat and their Culture Section would pick up one person from the employees of the U.S. Embassy to replace him. I have always enjoyed the work of the Cultural Section because the main task is cultural exchanges between China and the United States. I love working in this range. I was embarrassed to talk to Commercial Counsellor Richard Johnston saying I wanted to change jobs to work for the Culture Section. I asked him whether I could go to be interviewed to be the chief translator they wanted. Unexpectedly, Mr. Johnston smiled and said, you know that we Americans respect a person's free choice. Although I don't want you to leave the Commercial Section, but I won't stop you because I respect your wishes. I could hardly believe what he said. It was too generous, and too moving. So, I went to the Culture Section for the interview. After a few minutes of talking to me, the cultural counsellor said, "we're glad you're willing to come and work here. Can you start next

Monday?" I said yes. But I need to ask the Commercial Counsellor. I went back to the office of the Commercial Section and knocked at the door of Mr. Johnston. I just said that the Cultural Section wanted me to go to work next Monday. He had the same smile and he said very kindly, "I already knew. The Cultural Counsellor just called me. Congratulations!"

That night, as soon as I got home, I saw Bingsheng's serious face. It turned out that the leader had already talked to him. They heard about my desire to move (I didn't have time to report to them yet) and disagreed. Bingsheng said that the leader asked him to persuade me to change my mind and go back to work in The Commercial Section. It was like a basin of cold water spilled on me. I asked why? He said the leader said there might be a bad impact. I said, what's the impact? This was an internal transfer. The counsellors in both sections agreed. I'm supposed to work at the Culture Section next Monday, how do I quit? Bingsheng said that the leaders were worried that everyone would say that Li Xianghui was too free and would go wherever she wanted. I said angrily that it wasn't their arrangement.

Yet Bingsheng persuaded me to accept the leader's idea. I could not think straight and I did not agree to withdraw. We were deadlocked. I was so disappointed that I didn't even eat dinner. Finally Bingsheng said, "You should think about it. If you persist in switching your job, what will be the result? How will it affect me in my future work? I could not imagine what kind of actions they would take towards me." Obey or disobey-that is the question. "Disobey the leader"- once this big hat is buckled on a person, he/she is doomed! After a weekend of thinking, I had to compromise. According to the leader's suggestion, I went to Mr. Johnston, the Commercial Counselor, on Monday and said, "About the transfer, I went home and told my husband but he did not agree. The reason was that I worked very well in The Commercial Section and I would have to start from scratch if I switched to The Culture Section. So, I don't want to go to there now."

I was saying this to Mr. Johnston against my will and followed what the leader had told me. I felt as if I was forcing myself to swallow what I had just spit out. It was as disgusting as swallowing a fly. It also looked like I punched myself in the face with my own hand. Otherwise, what would be my options? I told Mr. Johnston a lie. He still had that smiling face and said, "That's great. Welcome back."

Walking out of his office, I didn't know whether to be happy or sad. This incident also laid a hidden danger for me when I came to the United States later. I was considered "an important person" in the Diplomatic Service Bureau, or maybe a person with a special assignment who was placed in the Commercial Section.

In 1987 I arrived at the University of San Francisco for a little more than a month. I received a phone call from the FBI. They followed me for years and found out that I was not interested in politics at all and had no special assignments, so they let me go.

Since the job switch failed, I felt that I was no more than a chess piece. I had no legs, thus I couldn't work. I had no wings, thus I could not fly. I could only passively live at the mercy of others. I deeply realized that no matter what a person's subjective wish was, objectively he/she could never jump over the circle others put around them. I also saw that Bingsheng was indeed a good husband who was considerate of me, understood me, and helped me in every aspect. My willfulness would have bad consequences for both of us. I had to swallow my complaints and grievances. But I was born a peacock, a bird who loves freedom. My soul refused to live in a cage. I have in my blood the genes of Manchu women rebelling against injustice. All those experiences planted the seeds for me to leave the Diplomatic

Service Bureau. With China's policy of opening doors to the outside world, the wind of studying abroad was getting stronger and stronger. One of my college schoolmates left her college teaching position to study at San Francisco State University. With her instigation and help, and with Bingsheng's consent (he knew that I was not happy working in the Service Bureau), I resolutely decided to leave this envied position, left Bingsheng and my lovely nine year-old daughter behind for what I thought would be only a year at that time. I flew to San Francisco, which was a place I had only seen occasionally in movies.

There was also an unexplainable happening in our life. I later seemed to find the answer in the confusion of why Bingsheng and I could not go to the end as a husband and wife. That is Providence and Destiny. There was no way we could get rid of it. Here's what happened. After I got my U.S. visa (I applied twice before it was approved), I started shopping a plane ticket. It was July 1987. Bingsheng was sent to the United Kingdom for a visit (at that time he had been transferred to the Education Department of the Diplomatic Service Bureau to train English speakers). His schedule of returning to Beijing was not certain. I left Beijing on July 13, 1987. It was a Friday. 13 and it was considered unlucky numbers for Americans. No wonder I couldn't book a ticket for another date. Bingsheng flew back to Beijing the next day, July 14. I was thinking, how did it happen? God didn't give the two of us a chance to bid each other farewell. Maybe God was afraid that we would be too sad to say goodbye in person. We didn't see each other until 5 years later!

I asked several masters why we, a loving couple, did not last to the end. A Taoist master said, "The connection of our two have ended. It is Karma..." Another Buddhist master said, "This is a fateful thing, no one can change it, even if you didn't go abroad, there will be a marriage change...." In the face of fate, why are we people so helpless? No one can refuse the destiny. Is it everything arranged?

Chapter 9

Love with My Second Husband

Now let me write about these inseparable "gentlemen" in my life. The reason why I am a brilliant woman in the eyes of my friends today is because of these gentlemen's sunshine. Marriage is a legal contract determined by people, but love is the energy of a finite life that cannot disappear in the infinite universe. Contracts make people live in peace, but it is the energy of nature that drives the wheels of life. Life is colorful. My Prince Charming, Bingsheng nick name Ice, not only gave me a wonderful family and the fruit of our love, a gentle, elegant, beautiful inside and out, intelligent, daughter Nancy; but also gave me a talented, versatile grandson Aaron, and lively and lovely granddaughter, Audrey. The three of them are the joy, pride, and motivation in my life. All three have Bingsheng's genes. I have given all my energy to them and love them in every way.

Bingsheng and I were classmates when we were teenagers. When we became boy and girl friends, the deep affection and friendship were vivid in my mind. When we were a loving couple, and when we were husband and wife, all the good times were unforgettable. The inner torment and pain after our breakup lasted for a long time. This irreparable regret and sadness left me heartbroken, uneasy, and haunted. My family was also sorry and worried about both of us. Every time my close friend Zhou Yulian saw me, she always said, "How did you two end up separated while not long ago you two were so affectionate? IfI had magic power, I would definitely let you both get back together like in the past...." Yes, over the years, I can imagine how difficult it is to carry life alone by himself. Bingsheng had suffered indescribable pain alone day and night! He is truly a manly husband! How could I not admire him? No one can appreciate better than me what he has suffered and how difficult the road he has traveled. His hard life is also my boundless sea of suffering.

On July 14 it was Bing-sheng's 75th birthday. As an old saying goes, "It is rare for people to live up to 70." For more than thirty years, the two of us had met several times on various occasions, and there were always others present, and even our polite greetings were infrequent. I subconsciously felt that I should do something no matter what his attitude would be. I had to sincerely communicate with him, talk to him from my heart, and will have no regrets in this life. I was willing to open that closed screen and give friends and family a little comfort. It was also like sweeping away the dark clouds in my heart. I was willing to send greetings, to send a touch of warmth to the heart that has been hurt for so many years. Hopefully there would be no more regrets.

I resolutely wrote this letter to him. Ice (his English name),

July 14 is your 75th birthday. Let me wish you good health and longevity here. Thank you for giving me a good daughter.

We have a pair of smart and lovely grandchildren. They stand out, and in them shine the roots of your goodness, intelligence, wisdom, and good genes. They also lived up to my expectation after all my hard work and dedication to them over the years. Now they appear as the most beautiful flowers bloom in the garden of our lives. All along, there were words that weighed on my heart. I didn't know how to say them to you. Without you, I almost lost my life. The happenings of the world are not subject to man's will. Up to now, I only sincerely hope that you will be healthy after experiencing the hardship of the past years. Nancy's growth, success, and her pair of angels are our rainbow. I sincerely hope that we can get along well and melt that piece of ice in our daughter's heart. On the occasion of your birthday, I will tell you what is in my heart and hopefully make up for the regret of not communicating with you for so many years. Right or wrong, a thousand words, just want to say Hello. You are a gentleman, a benefactor who has fulfilled me in so many ways. Let's live a good and healthy life. I hope we can share the good life of our children.

Here I send you eternal blessings. Happy birthday!

When he received my message, he quickly echoed it, also in English, "Thanks a lot. Bygones are gone with the wind."

Later last year I sent him a video of our granddaughter playing the piano, and he was overjoyed to see how wonderful our third generation had come along.

Believing in the success of our children will make us both happy for the rest of our lives. For many years, I have been sad, silently bearing blame, hiding the pain in my heart, and tried smiling to meet the future life and reality of every day. I seem to be reborn, a Nirvana Rebirth! The long river of years is flowing quietly, and the acquaintance, encounter, love, are beyond our mortal control. However, love with my first husband is never forgotten.

The second gentleman in my life was Eugene Olson, or Gene for short. He is ten years older than me. According to the Chinese lunar calendar, he was born in the year of the pig, and according to the constellation, he is a Libra. He was polite, kind, gentle, knowledgeable and understanding. I learned many things from him.

His specialty was painting, and he not only often took me to museums in San Francisco to see a wide variety of exhibitions or helped me understand Western history, culture, religion, painting, and music, but also introduced to me all the movie stars in Hollywood movies. I took him back to Beijing in 2006. My family members all called him Mr. Gene. I think the name Gene (金 fits him too well.) In Chinese the pronunciation of Gene means Gold. He does have a heart of good, pure gold. My Chinese family members all call him Mr. Gold.

Gene is a tall man of 6 feet. His blue eyes are always full of kindness and friendliness. He never says anything bad of anyone, and even if others bullied him and obviously took advantage of him, he would not say a word, as if he did not know how to get angry. His father was full-blood Norwegian and his mother was full-blood Irish. It can be seen that he mainly inherited the kindness, sincerity and indisputable character of the Norse people. No matter what happened, he always looked forward with optimism and hope. He said that looking forward always gives hope and light. Gene's love exudes an energy. Eighteen years into his marriage, I've never heard him say anything hurtful about anyone, and he has never been picky or jealous of anyone. I learned a lot of good qualities from him.

His love for me was sometimes like that of a loving father, sometimes like a brother in brotherhood. Gene's kindness and unconditional fatherly love and dedication, magnanimous and meticulous care, touched me deeply. He treated my daughter Nancy as his own daughter. He acted as a loving father, and a close friend, and for more than ten years helped me cultivate my daughter into an outstanding graduate of the Engineering Department of the University of California at Berkeley. On the brink and in the midst of my life's pain, he accompanied me and helped bring me back to life. Love is the power of the soul; love is the light of the spirit; the expression and action of kindness. I am grateful to him for the rest of my life. I never forget.

After years of separation from him, my girlfriend always mentioned to me a conversation she had with Gene. She said, "One time, when I went to your house for a party, I saw with my own eyes that he had ironed all the clothes he had washed for you and put them in a drawer." I said, "You're such a good husband."

Gene said, 'Tm very happy to do something for her as long as she lets me love her."

My girlfriend told me that she was so touched to hear that. She is very glad that I had such a husband who loves me. While revising my autobiography, I received a thick book that Gene had recently completed, titled "The Wonderful Life of Gene Olson and His Family." What a coincidence that he was also recalling his own life, using many wonderful photos, a memorial to life itself. The two of us were really well matched. We were both summing up our lives with our hearts and souls remembering the good life we spent together. In his memoir, he uses many photographs to introduce readers to his life and family background, from childhood to adulthood.

Gene received the degree of Bachelor of Science from Portland State College, and the degree of Master of Science in Teaching, majoring in painting. He was the director of the Department of Culture and Sports in Concord, California, USA. When he worked there, he organized countless large and small theatrical performances and sports activities, and also met many celebrities.

Everyone's life is accompanied by happiness, sadness, and pain cannot be avoided, but good people are offering their best love for everyone. In Gene's book there is special page for Nancy. One can clearly see that Nancy is also a flower in his heart. In the process of helping me to cultivate Nancy's growth, he made an indelible contribution. Now, Nancy, including her two children, are in regular contact with Gene. In the pictures of our lives together and the places we had been, he noted the locations. He also made several pages for me. There wasn't a single picture of us without a smile on our faces. On the last page of the book, Gene wrote with a thick pen on the photograph, "Lydia, Thank you for a great life. Gene Olson 2022."

Yes, the hearts of good people only record the good. The more I wrote, the more I felt that I was so lucky. The second husband, whom I left later, never resented me, but blessed my new life. My happiness is his happiness. How selfless he was! His incomparable kindness and blessing once again confirmed that kindness is the best Feng Shui in the world. His kindness is a rainbow shining every day. How can I not be touched? I met such a great man in this life. It's a continual blessing on my life.

In the face of love, I was a failing elementary school student, but life is also a learning process. Spending time with Gene made me feel deeply that he was my mentor, and he taught me kindness and love. Because of his dedication over the years, he planted the most beautiful flowers in the garden of life. Although we can't accompany each other for the rest of our lives, his character which has always been beautiful and kind to others, has created our rare friendship today, the most beautiful love and the highest realm under the rainbow.

Chapter 10

The Turning Point in Life

Overall, I'm one of the lucky ones. Most self-funded international students or immigrants from mainland China had to work first, and most of them do manual labor or service in restaurants. Before I came to the United States, I already had work lined up as an office manager. My college schoolmate also helped me find a live-in position in an American family. I didn't have to pay food or board but no salary. My job was to baby-sit two boys on weekends, one was nine and the other was five. The couple could go out and party with friends, watch movies, etc.

Soon an American lawyer I had helped in Beijing who knew I was in San Francisco called me to help his law firm to do some translation work. So, my income was considerable because there was no cost for room or board. When I talked to the director of the International Student Division at San Francisco State University about my desire to invite my husband and daughter in China to visit the United States, he didn't say a word and immediately printed me an invitation letter. How I wished them to see the America I had discovered with their own eyes. I was very disappointed to wait for an answer for more than a month and received a rejection answer. The head of the Diplomatic Service Bureau said that he could approve me to extend my studies for another year, but Bingsheng could not get a passport, which meant that he was not allowed to come to the United States to see me!

Actually, they took him as an "hostage." They were afraid that our family of three would not go back after they came to the United States. The originally loving husband and wife, a harmonious family of three, seemed to have suddenly suffered a heavy downpour and was soaked. Bingsheng saw that our daughter missed me day and night, he applied again to approve my daughter come to visit me. The authority agreed and Bingsheng sent our daughter to the airport and entrusted a nice China airline attendant to chaperon Nancy to San Francisco. Our ten-year-old daughter bravely boarded the plane and flew alone from Beijing to San Francisco airport. I haven't seen my daughter for a year and a half. When I saw her walk out, I was so excited and happy that I took her in my arms at once. No matter what might happen in the future, I would never leave my daughter again!

For my precious daughter Wang Xiao-nan, Nancy, I would sacrifice everything for her. To welcome my daughter to come to the United States, I bought a new car. I sent her to school every day and then went to my work, and then picked her up. One year-and-a-half separation of mother and daughter was finally over. In the middle of the night, watching my lovely daughter sleeping sweetly beside me, I couldn't help but hold her in my arms. I kissed her sweet little face, touched her plum little feet. I look forward to the day when Ice could come and reunited with us.

Whoever expected a succession of events would catch me off guard like a thunderbolt on a sunny day? First, I took Nancy to Disneyland and we had such a good time. On the way back, my new car was hit by two Mexican guys and had to be towed away. Fortunately, Nancy were blessed and did not get hurt seriously. Second, the consulting firm I worked in San Francisco decided to move their office to Shanghai.

Mr. Gene Olson was a good friend of mine then. We were introduced to know each other by Rena who asked me whether I could help her friend Gene to sell some used medical instruments to China. To put the long story short, Gene and I became good friends. He was very impressed by my courage to leave China to live in a new world successfully. He learned on the phone that I had a car accident and was very worried. He called from Crescent City to my good friend Rena who worked in San Francisco and asked her to help me deal with insurance for the car accident. Coincidentally, when Gene called Rena, I was sitting in Rena's office. I did not have a chance to tell Rena about my car accident yet. Seeing Rena holding the phone in her hand and looking at me with wide eyes I knew Gene must be telling her my car accident. After she talked to Gene, I told her what happened on our way back from Disneyland. She was relieved that she saw my daughter and I were all right. Later on, Gene called me offering Nancy and I rest in his place for a while and wait for the settlement of my car insurance to handle the issue. He drove down and picked me up and my daughter to Crescent City, a small seaside city in northern California where he worked as the Executive Director of Del Norte County Senior Center. The pristine forest is nestled against the beautiful Pacific Sea. I am grateful for the help he gave me and Nancy in a critical moment.

That year, 1989, on June 4th, Tiananmen Incident occurred in China. What I saw on American television was that bleeding students were pulled by tricycles to hospitals. The commentators said they were shot by Chinese army or ran over by tanks. On the contrary, what Bingsheng saw on Chinese television was how students obstructed traffic and normal civic life, soldiers were beaten, and cars were burned. Nancy asked her father when he called us on the phone, "What happened to the students of Tiananmen?" I was angrily criticized by Bingsheng, "How did you teach Nancy?" Misunderstandings and rumors deepened the gap between me and Bingsheng and pushed me into an abyss of helplessness. When I wrote to him and told him that I didn't want my daughter to grow up under that system. I wanted Nancy to enjoy the freedom here. He wrote back angrily to me, "You can stay there and enjoy your freedom and give back my daughter!" He also said, "Grandparents missed Nancy so much that they got sick and you are fully responsible for its consequences!" Later, he also sent me an "order" in large characters: Order of a divorce! I saw at our originally happy family about to break up. Thinking that my in-laws and their daughters and son were very close to me and our Li family's all liked and respected for Bingsheng, I really didn't know what to do. Leave the U.S. going back to China? I discussed with Nancy,

"Otherwise let's go back to Beijing?" What I never expected was that Nancy cried and said to me, "I won't go back! I can't keep up with my homework, besides, Xiaolan (her aunt's second daughter) will be better than me and she will laugh at me."

Every day, I suffered between my innocent daughter and the helpless me: leaving or not , returning home or staying in the United States. I had no one to talk to or discuss things with. Every day, I wandered on the seashore of the Pacific Ocean in Crescent City, looking at the motherland six thousand miles on the other side of the ocean. I was completely lost. Tears filled in my eyes and pains filled in my heart. There was no one to talk to, and there was nowhere to turn to. I spent countless sleepless nights. Later, when I met Bingsheng's elder sister in Portland, Oregon, she told me that when my mother-in-law found out Bingsheng and I were "fighting," she wrote me a letter to teach me that people will always have some contradictions in middle age. I should be considerate of Bingsheng's situation, and take Nancy back to China as soon as possible. Sister also said, "If you read mother's letter, you might change your decision." But the letter that my mother-in-law asked Bing-sheng to mail to me never came-he never mailed it.

Originally, I didn't want to write these painful details, but why didn't Bingsheng and I, who were originally a loving couple that everyone envied, go on to remain a happy family? Is it true that people have come to the conclusion that I had an affair and abandoned him? I once wrote to Bingsheng that I had a car accident and lost my job. I stayed at a friend's house for a while.

I didn't want to divorce him at all because I loved him. His reply was, "You don't deserve to talk about love!"

This not only greatly broke my heart, but also made me suspect that he had a girl friend in Beijing and did not love me anymore. I certainly understood his irritation.

Later, I heard that my "Chinese friend" in the United States returned to Beijing to report to the director of the Diplomatic Service Bureau where I worked that I had a boyfriend in the United States. The director had a talk with Bingsheng and indicted he should divorce me, otherwise his political future would be ruined. Bingsheng was a popular figure and had a very high esteem in the Diplomatic Service Bureau. Now his wife had gone to the United States and did not come back because she found a foreign boyfriend. She betrayed the motherland as well as betrayed her husband. His face was lost thoroughly. An American officer at the U.S. Visa Service of the U.S. Embassy in Beijing heard that I was not going back to China angrily said that he would not issue any visas to any service bureau personnel who requested to go to the U.S. I really became the black sheep

Bingsheng used to go to the downstairs of our diplomatic

residence in the embassy district every night to play poker or chess with our neighbors (both of which he was a master) and because of my reasons, he stayed in the house and did not go out anymore. When I heard about this later, I really hated myself.

I asked Mr. Gao Peng, the wife of Mr. Wang Nai, president of Peili University (The first private university in Beijing where I taught English in my spare time in the 80s. The couple came to California to babysit the children for their daughter and we became close friends) went back to Beijing to speak to Bingsheng about my return to China to see what his attitude was. Teacher Gao brought back the words: Bing-sheng said, "She is a bird that flew out of the cage. If you let the bird fly back into the cage, will she be happy? If she comes back for the sake of me but will not be happy in the future, I don't want to take on that responsibility." He also said, "If the broken mirror is reunion, the crack will remain there forever. Tell her not to come back." Readers, what would you feel hearing these answers? Can I not cry? I've caused him so much pain! Teacher Gao advised me, "I don't think you need to hesitate anymore; people won't only love one person in their lives. You'd better give up Bingsheng for the sake of the future of your daughter."

Gene was really like a pearl in my life. His silent companionship and selfless help held up an umbrella for me to shield me from the wind and rain when I was most helpless and in pain. He expected no return, had no expectations, just an incomparable understanding of me and unconditional love. He gave me a safe haven. When I told him that Bingsheng and I had a conflict, he also said, "You Chinese handle things differently from us Americans. According to what I heard, you two are a kind couple and still in love. When you are separated, you should tell each other how you miss and love each other but not complain about each other." He also sincerely told me that I could make my own decision. "If you have to take Nancy back to China, I will miss you, but I absolutely respect your choice; If you decide to stay in the U.S., I'll help you raise Nancy." I was between two people: one angry and cold; one gentle and kind, without any demands or expectations. If you were me, what would you do?

After thinking about it and discussing it with my friends at home and abroad, I decided to stay. My younger sister went through the divorce procedures with Bingsheng on my behalf in Beijing. The pain and suffering of both of us lasted for many years, and even sent us to the death door in a different way: Bing sheng was so depressed that his immune system declined. He was admitted to Beijing Hospital but the high fever did not go away for days. His doctor issued a medical crisis notice. I also had cancer out of depression. Fortunately, Yama confiscated us and sent us back to our relatives and friends. Neither of us died. Maybe God also hurt and pitied us both.

Love, no matter in which country, what cultural background, what kind of world view, whether rich or poor, is like the sun and everyone yearns for that warmth. But on the other hand, love is like also a sword. She can pierce you mercilessly! Love, what a charming and beautiful word, a state of mind, a feeling, an inexplicable, unclear thing, so that millions of people experienced its joy, excitement, tears, blood, sleepless nights, for it is unforgettable. One can sacrifice everything for it, and it pains all men and it hurts all women. Each person's experience is different because the country is different, the cultural background is different, the way of thinking is different, therefore, there will be different explanations, interpretations and conclusions.

Generally speaking, Chinese's understanding of love is to love, to stay together, to be loyal, to have the same feelings. To go to the next level is to sacrifice everything for each other. In the Western world, such as the United States, love is about appreciating your appearance, your character, and your inner feelings. It can be permanent, or it can be "changing with each passing day" (some exaggeration). It can be because of one thing that you fall in love with, or it can be because one thing he or she doesn't love you anymore. Few people think love is eternal. Once there is a change, "there is a reason," most people's attitude is "then I will not hang on to it, and let you go, I will find new love." The next level is "as long as you are happy, I can fulfill you."

I think love is a combination of spirit, soul and flesh. It is the most beautiful emotion in the world, from which you can draw infinite energy, but also mixed with pains. It means understanding, heartache, compromise, dedication and sacrifice of yourself. It can make you cry and bleed. Escaping into Buddhism and away from the world may also be a way of escaping the trouble of falling in love.

I have slowly come to realize that some people's kindness may not be rewarded in this life, but I firmly believe that their great and selfless love is brilliant and will be rewarded in the next life. A better ending and love await. My three husbands were highly cultivated and loved me selfishly. Not only do I feel very happy to be able to share 16 years of happy life with each of them, but I have always respected, appreciated, and remembered them. Love is a complex emotion that is difficult to articulate in words. They perfected my soul. So far, I have maintained respectful and friendly contact with them both. This is a situation that many people cannot imagine and cannot comprehend . I have expressed my feelings and gratitude to them in different ways, and I have said the same thing to my friends and family.

Someone once asked me bluntly: What is the use of how highly you think of them now? In fact you are "turning your back" on them. I don't want to excuse myself anymore. Love is subtle and it's multi-faceted. In a way, I'm a selfish Manchu woman centered upon myself.

However, in many cases, under the impact of politics and culture in different countries, I am also involuntarily forced to do what I need to do. I feel that it is the arrangement of the divine, the mandate of fate.

Although I came to the United States for a few years, I seemed to be in good shape. My work, studies, and life were relatively smooth. However, the sad thing that made me most miserable is that I missed my family, my relatives at home! The taste of biting your soul that can't be expressed to anyone is so uncomfortable. I worked in two companies during the day from Monday to Friday and attended classes at school from 7 to 10 o'clock in the evening. I was busy, so busy that I had no time to be homesick. But on weekends, it's like I lost my soul.

I didn't know if my daughter Nancy and her father went back to Grandma Xizhimen's house to visit, or what they were doing at my own house in Sanlitun. At that time, there was no phone at home, no e-mail, and a letter took more than ten days to arrive. I missed them so much that tears streamed down my cheeks, but I had nobody to talk to. I had to secretly swallow the pain. So here, I want to persuade parents who want their children to go abroad, or people who want to go abroad, to think twice. "A thousand days at home are always good, while everything is difficult when you leave home." Especially the feel of homesickness and the taste of missing family are not worth leaving home. I came to the United States as an IAP-66, self funded visiting scholar. According to the immigration laws of the United States, visiting scholars must return home for two years before they can re-enter the United States. I know that once I go back and then coming back will be almost impossible.

My personal experience made me later become a "big sister Li" who could patiently listen to others talk about their hesitations, contradictions, pains because I know what a person needs when he/

she spirals into the circle of life's problems, especially when they are suffering from emotional pains. So no matter where I live, I have friends who confide in me about their inner worlds. Even if I'm just a listener, I make them feel a little more comfortable and relieved. I feel that my life has a renewed value.

Chapter 11

Life in Crescent City

I was an IAP-66 Visiting Scholar. Because President Bush issued a presidential amnesty after June 4th incident happened in Beijing, Chinese IAP students who came to the United States before June 4, 1989, were exempt from the requirement of returning to China for two years and then were allowed to re enter the United States. They could apply for a long-term residence green card. My relationship with Bingsheng dropped to zero. If Gene and I went through the marriage procedures, then I would be double insured to stay in the U. S. So we got married, which ensured Nancy and I could legally stay in the U.S. Crescent City had a population of just over three thousand people among them , eight Chinese. Almost everyone knows each other there. Nancy's adaptability was amazing. Soon she was able to speak English without any accent. I went to attend a parent-teacher meeting. Her teacher told me, "Your daughter is a very unusual girl. Although her English expression ability is limited, but she understands the words of the teacher and her classmates very quickly. Even if she does not fully understand, she always smiles. Everyone likes her as a lovely Chinese doll. Her math was surprisingly good. She could teach math to the whole class." A year later, Nancy went from elementary school to junior high school. By the end of the first semester, she had already ranked the best in her school. When she graduated from junior high school, she and another American classmate tied for the first place in the school. Nancy Wang had become a Chinese doll that everyone knew and loved. Watching her blossoming like a flower, my heart was blossoming too. Only there was that dark shadow which won't leave me-her father was stuck in Beijing, China.

My daughter and I also made a lot of American friends. We attended local musicals, drama performances. Our activities included quartet choirs on Mondays, international folk dance on Tuesdays, ballet practice on Wednesdays and Fridays. I also attended the senior Tennis Club in Brookings, Oregon on Monday, Wednesday, and Friday mornings. Every Chinese New Year, I invited a few American friends to come to our house to enjoy Chinese dumplings. Nancy accompanied me on the piano, and I sang Chinese folk songs to them. Gene put on the Chinese outfit I bought for him, dressed up as a waiter, welcomed the guests, and poured wine for everyone. The Chinese New Year atmosphere created by Nancy and I had resolved some of our homesickness. There were no Chinese shops around us, not even a Chinese calendar. I didn't even know which day would be Moon Festival. After inquiring about the date of the Chinese holidays, I always invited American friends to come to our home, cooked them Chinese food, and introduced Chinese culture.

The principal of a local elementary school also invited me to her school and asked American elementary school students to kowtow to me and pay homage to Chinese New Year. At that time (80s, 90s), the vast majority of Americans did not understand China. Many people thought that China was not only far away from America in terms of distance but also had no idea about the culture or unpredictable life. Their impression of China was that people there were very poor and the government was an oppressive dictatorship. However, they were curious about China and they wanted to know what a big country in the distance was like and how people's lives were.

A local non-profit organization organized cultural and artistic classes for local primary and secondary schools. The director asked me if I could open a Chinese culture class in local school district. I appreciated her thinking and supported her suggestion. I also thought that this would be a good opportunity to introduce to the children of the United States and their parents of my mysterious country in the Far East. After discussing with the director, I taught several courses: "Speaking Chinese", "Writing Chinese Characters", "Taiji Basic Skills", "Taiji Sword" and so on. Every semester, local teachers from more than 20 classes signed up for my Chinese Cultural classes. The youngest were first-grade elementary school students and the oldest were teenage students of junior high school.

On the first day of the class, I hung a map of China on the blackboard of the classroom introducing China's geographical location, population and my birthplace, the great and brilliant capital, Beijing. A Beijing picture album which I brought to the United States from China introduced Beijing's royal gardens, Forbidden City, Summer Palace, Winter Palace, Temple of Heaven, Temple of Earth, Dr. Sen Yensen Park, Tiananmen Square, Xiangshan, Biyun Temple, Great Wall, etc. Teachers and students were all fascinated. They never dreamed that China was such a beautiful and magical place. I was encouraged and excited by the class I went to, where the teachers and students were not only curious, but also full of joy and eagerness. They wrote Chinese characters seriously and learned Tai Chi movements happily. Later, I also opened a calligraphy class in junior high school to teaching them writing Chinese characters with Chinese ink and brushes. I translated everyone's English name into Chinese and explained to them the Chinese meaning of each character. They were overjoyed to be able to write their own names in Chinese!

July 4 of each year was Independence Day in the U. S.. In

addition to large parades, the cultural center organized exhibitions of artwork and paintings. Artists rent a booth to display and sell their own artwork. Gene always rented a booth to display his paintings of various boats. Gene suggested that I add a table next to his booth to write people's names in Chinese using the cardboard he made for me. I charge $5 per person. Sometimes there were lines waiting. They were surprised and happy when they saw that their names could be pronounced and written in Chinese characters. In Crescent City, a small coastal town in the far north of California, in the halls of the cultural center that were full of western paintings and various works of art, my small table with ink and brush was very special. It was like a foreign wind blowing into the hearts of Americans.

I taught American children about Chinese culture at Crescent City schools. The Chinese calligraphy on the wall in the picture was given to me by Ye Shengbao, the younger brother of my brother-in-law, before I left Beijing for the United States. The two of us are one year apart, and his ping-pong skill and Peking Opera singing are close to professional level. Unfortunately, when the two of us were in Beijing, we were both busy far and we could not have more exchanges as we wished. Luckily, when I returned to Beijing in the fall of 2017, he accompanied me a to play table-tennis and sing Peking Opera. Now 6,000 miles away, on the other side of the ocean and the epidemic, it is difficult to meet. I went back to Beijing in 2018 again and I had a wonderful time in the table tennis club and Peking opera group he was the leader. Unfortunately he passed away during Covid period before my book was published.

Later, the head of the Crescent City Recreation Department asked me to start a Tai Chi class at their gymnasium. I didn't expect the people who signed up my class were very enthusiastic. At many local celebration occasions, I was invited to perform such as local high school graduation ceremonies, women's clubs, county fairs, senior centers and local cultural activities at different times and in different places. I have performed 24 styles of Tai Chi, 32 styles of Tai Chi Sword, Mulan single fan dancing, Mulan double fan dancing, Chinese folk dance, Chinese folk songs and so on. Next to the lush Pacific Ocean in that primitive redwood forest, a small city not known by many and no Chinese culture, when the beautiful music of "Spring River with Flowers under the Moon Night" and "Butterfly Lovers" were played in the loudspeaker, it attracted the curiosity and attention of local residents and people who came for vacation from all directions. I put on my traditional Chinese costumes and performed for them gracefully. As a Chinese, I felt very proud to be able to share my knowledge with local Americans in a small coastal city on the other side of the Pacific Ocean.

When I taught adults Chinese and Tai Chi, I found that my students were so fond of Asian cultures. They were not only engaged in learning but also full of respect for me. I had established a very harmonious teacher-student relationship with them. Some of them had become my friends. A student and friend, a Chinese fan, who had been to China many times once asked me, "You have so many friends and relatives in China, besides there are so many delicious foods in China. You are not an adult who grew up in the United States, but you chose to stay here. Do you miss them? Do you feel lonely in your heart?" I said, "I do miss my friends and family and all kinds of Chinese food, but my heart and my mind are filled with Chinese culture, knowledge and history. My heart is full and I feel rich spiritually." She smiled and nodded her head with approval expression. Every time something happened in China, she liked to talk to me about it. Whoever said that China was not good, she would argue with them.

Although I chose to stay in the United States, the seeds of

Chinese culture were deeply planted in my blood. That is my spiritual food; that is my root; that is what makes me never forget that I am a Chinese and be proud of it. I think Chinese people all over the world are like this. Whenever they hear Chinese songs, see Chinese dances, Peking opera, acrobatics, no matter when and where, they are overjoyed and feel closer to the motherland. When I found that my daughter Nancy had been in the U.S. for three years but her Chinese started to get rusty, I took her back to Beijing in 1992. Bingsheng and I decided to let Nancy return to the third grade of junior high school of Beijing No. 55 Middle School. Even though she went through a difficult ordeal, this decision benefited her greatly for her later life and work. Now she has been insisting that her two children take Chinese classes three times a week after normal school hours. Whenever I hear them speaking authentic English and Chinese, my heart is filled with joy. They are lucky to have a pair of parents who not provide enough materials for then but also care deeply about their academic study and culture heritage. The two kids have taken classes of piano, vocal music, painting, football, basketball, tennis, golf, fencing, swimming, skiing, rowing, Chinese, Japanese. I'm very proud of them. When my English version of biography is to be published this year my grandson will be in George Washington University.

After Nancy returned from Beijing, she attended high school in Crescent City, California. In addition to the love of her father in Beijing, Nancy also received a lot of fatherly love from Gene in America. In addition to becoming an all-around student at the school, Nancy took ballet classes from local dance school, a member of high school tennis team and also participated in the high school speech and debate team. In successive lectures on and off campus, the trophies she received at the speech tournaments and debates occupied the whole top of the piano.

The topic of her first speech was "The Great Wall of China." After won the first round locally, she had to go to San Francisco State University to participate in a state level competition. I also drove 350 miles to S.F. to cheer her up. After several rounds of competition, a list of six students in the final was posted on the wall of the hallway. Both my daughter and I saw Nancy Wang's name on the list. Nancy smiled so happily that she could not close her month. I was so excited that I ran back to my car and started to cry before I could sit down.

Since coming to the United States, I went through ups and downs, worked hard, paid great attention to watch almost every minute for Nancy's safety and to be sure that she feels no less than any other child. In order to give her the opportunity to study in the United States, I was literality being charged with the crime of betraying the motherland and betraying my husband. I lost my dear husband; lost my prestigious job in Beijing; lost my warm and happy family. Suddenly, Nancy's success was boiling my heart. Everything I lost hurt my heart. What I sacrificed was not in vain. Nancy had stepped onto the track of success. The intricate feelings in my heart was indescribable. Those who had no personal experience like mine would not be able to understand my crying was also a kind of venting. Up to today, I still haven't told my daughter that the first time she won the speech final why I ran back to the car and why I cried.

I hope that one day, when she reads my autobiography, she will understand a mother's pain, grievances, bitterness, and excitement. Nancy became the main force of the debate team and was selected to attend the summer speech and debate training courses at the University of Berkeley and Stanford University. She was also the main force of Del Norte high school tennis team at the time, and the only Chinese girl in the amateur ballet school. Whenever Nancy performed on stage, Gene and I went to the theatre early in order to find a better place to video her. Once I happened to see tears in Gene's eyes when he watched Nancy performing on stage. After we arrived at home, I asked him why he was in tears. He said movingly that Nancy was dancing so beautifully. None of those American girls were as graceful and elegant as she was. I proudly said that it was in her genes.

I also found a piano teacher and a viola professor to teach Nancy. Her life was full of positive energy outside the three dimensional world. She is busy. The joy and constant improvement of high-quality cultural edification were like sunshine and rain bathing her healthily and thrivingly. During those days, Gene did his best to help me cultivate Nancy's talents in all aspects. Every morning Gene took her to school. I picked her up in the afternoon. She communicate with Gene about everything. Maybe I was in menopause, my temper was unstable, and I couldn't control the nameless fire from within. If I wanted to know anything about Nancy, for example, the details of the speech competition, how many prizes she won, and the details of the game she played on the tennis team, I have to hear from Gene. Thanks for Gene that Nancy had a family member to confide and communicate. When she graduated from Del Norte high school, three of the universities she applied admitted her, but she did not say anything. Finally the acceptance letter from the Chemistry Department of University of Berkeley came. She had a big smile on her face, The whole school was cheering. She was the only student admitted to Berkeley from remote Crescent City in years. At the high school graduation ceremony, Nancy received awards from more than a dozen different organizations, with prize money of more than 55,000 US dollars. That day was the happiest day she had ever been in the United States. Of course, my heart was filled with joy.

Chapter 12

My Endeavour

After moving from San Francisco to Crescent City, I learned to use a computer at a local aviation mapping company to calculate the timber company's logging output and draw maps. Working in two shifts, I had to stare at the plotter's screen to do the job, and the working environment was unpleasant, so I decided to go back to school to study for a master's degree in English. With a master's degree, jobs are easier to find, besides, one was eligible to work as a teacher either at community college or at a state university. In our area, there was only one university which offered master's degrees. It was called Humboldt State University, 78 miles from Crescent City. To pursue a master's degree in English, leaving home at 6 a.m. three days a week and returning home at 11 p.m. was very challenging. The master English classes were always scheduled in the evenings to facilitate students who worked during daytime. Driving that far I thought I might as well stay for the whole day. So I signed up for various classes.

What made me thrilled was that after you paid a certain amount of tuition, you could select any course. I took advantage of the opportunity to sign up for tennis lessons, vocal lessons, piano lessons, dance lessons, music appreciation lessons, etc.. I was always fascinated by literature, arts, and sports. Now it seemed that

I was blessed with a heavenly opportunity, allowing me to enjoy the spiritual wealth, but also get involved with the fields of culture and sports that were not easy for ordinary people to enter. I entered the four-dimensional, five-dimensional, and higher-dimensional worlds. The higher-dimensional world gave me boundless energy. I benefited from this greatly in my old age. The 78-mile journey took an hour and a half, with pristine redwood forests on one side of the road and the Pacific Ocean on the other side below the cliffs. I learned driving in the hilly downtown of San Francisco. So, I was not afraid of turns and hills. Highway 1 in the United States is very well built along the Pacific Ocean. The signs were also very clear and the speed limit was indicated for both turns and sharp turns. Sometimes the road went through the primeval forest. Sometimes it dashed from the mountain to the sea. The scenery was breathtaking. I regarded every journey to and from school as a special trip. I know that many people had to save money and take vacations to travel here. One day I would leave the beauty of this place and now I had to fully enjoy every bit of it.

To be on the safe side, Gene suggested I buy a used Lincoln sedan that was very comfortable and safe. I was listening to Western classical music that Gene recommended to me, such as the famous American singers Barbara Streisand, Bette Milder, Neil Diamond, Sarah Brightman, Canadian singer Celine Dion, and so on. Every morning when I started the engine, my audiovisual feast began. As I am writing this, I would like to thank my second husband, Mr. Gene Olson, for not only opening the door to the western world of painting, but also bringing me into the palace of Western music. I benefited immensely from this western culture. It was the spiritual food of my life.

When I started applying for a master's degree in English at Humbert University, Professor Turner, who was in charge of the master's application, initially doubted my English proficiency and suggested that I take two or three undergraduate English classes first. I signed up for the Shakespeare class he taught. At the end of the semester, several English professors who taught me said in unison that our English department had never recruited students whose native language was Chinese. They said my English comprehension and expression were beyond their expectations. I was an outstanding student. Professor Borough, whom I often debated with in class, later wrote me a letter of recommendation for applying to a Ph.D. degree program at Indiana University. He wrote that I was the best student he had taught for more than thirty years. When I took a vocal class, Professor Stannard of the Music Department worked with me to translate Chinese songs into English. I also performed "The Sea, My Hometown," a song that is well-known in China.

I studied in the English Department at Humbert University for five semesters and received a master's degree in English with two majors: teaching English writing, and English and American literature. This laid a solid foundation for me to be hired by four universities in the United States later on. During my study at the university, I also received three scholarships and was admitted to Indiana University as a candidate of Ph.D. student of Comparative Literature. At the same time, I also received funding for an internship at Indiana University for two months in the summer, and then officially attended the doctoral candidate's class when the semester began in September. In the summer of 1996, I went to Indiana University. It was a prestigious comprehensive university in the middle of the United States. Their sports department, especially basketball, is famous all over the world.

The Department of Music also attracts students from all over the world who want to study music. The Olympic-sized swimming pool became a must-visit place for me every day. The daily student free rehearsals at the concert hall were also a place I frequented. Violin, piano, and harp were my favorite instruments.

My Ph.D. tutor, a professor from Hong Kong, met with me once. He was going to the University of Hong Kong to have a sabbatical leave. An American professor in the English department who teaches English and American literature was responsible for guiding my summer studies. I read the works of several British literary grandmasters and discussed them with him. I also made a couple of Chinese friends in Indiana. Socializing with them, swimming together, playing tennis, eating, partying, helped me relieve my loneliness. I've been living in coastal California since I came to the U.S. in 1987 and haven't had a hot summer, but summer in Indiana reached 34 degrees Celsius every day! I also took part in tennis training twice a week. All of a sudden I dropped to 132 pounds.

Autumn is beautiful in Indiana. The red maple leaf forest looked like a mythical world. I was going to study for a Ph.D. in Comparative Literature. The topic was to compare the similarities and differences between my favorite classical Chinese novel Dream of the Red Chamber and the English literature of the same period. I was excited. I signed up for several required courses for the fall semester. At the same time, I applied for a Ph.D. study scholarship and a TA position (teaching assistant) for undergraduate students. Two or three weeks later, the school informed me that American Chinese students were not considered ethnic minorities there. So there was no scholarship for me. They granted me a student loan of eighteen thousand US dollars. In addition, the application for a teaching assistant in the Chinese department also failed because I was not a doctoral student in the Chinese department of the school. I belonged to the English department and they had to take care of the Ph.D. students in their Chinese department.

Since I came to the United States, I had paid my credit card in full every month. Now I would have a loan of eighteen thousand US dollars. I felt the pressure, which was very stressful. There were other reasons that I wanted to quit. One of the most important reasons was that my Ph.D. tutor was a professor who was born in Hong Kong and now was on a sabbatical leave for a year. I heard that he learned his Chinese at this university (Indiana University). "Can he tutor me on the classic novel Dream of the Red Chamber?" I doubted it. The only time I met him, he suggested that I should change my doctoral research topic to a more modern Chinese novel. It was 1996 then. I wasn't interested in contemporary fiction at all. In addition, Gene was alone in Crescent City, the northernmost part of California. My daughter Nancy just entered the University of Berkeley, and I was alone in Indiana with a big debt to manage. If they needed me, I didn't know ifI would be able to leave right away. Thinking all about these things, I decided to drop out of that program.

I was 51 years old and thought it didn't matter whether or not I could obtain a Ph.D. degree. Concentrating on raising my daughter and supporting her, were my duty. I was embarrassed to tell Professor Turner of Humbert University about my withdrawal from Indiana University. He was the mentor who accepted me as a Chinese student into the graduate program of the English Department. He also accompanied me on a tour to the University of Berkeley, Stanford University, the University of San Diego, including Indiana University (when I graduated from the graduate class in 1996, I received a pre-Doctoral bonus, but I had to be accompanied by a tutor to visit those four universities). The three English professors who taught me at Humbert University all wrote me very convincing letters of recommendation (three professorial letters of recommendation are required for PhD students). I felt that I had failed them. Professor Turner was very sorry. He said, in fact, "if you stick to it for another year, the next year will be much better."

My American dream was to see this beautiful country with my own eyes and let my husband and daughter experience everything this country had to offer. It was not necessary to get a master's or a doctoral degree. Here I turned my life's course away from serving my own personal goals, and towards service and caring for others. From Indiana I flew back to Crescent City, California. I felt like a fish that returned to the water. Later, I found the way I made decisions and handled things was emotional, not practical. I did not think much about the pros and cons. I always did what I wanted.

In May 2000, Nancy graduated from the University of Berkeley with a bachelor's degree in Industrial Engineering and Operation Research. I also taught English grammar fundamentals and writing classes for two years at the local Redwood College. Gene was preparing to retire at the end of that year. My friends on the East Coast, Ru Yan and her husband, made plans to visit Crescent City first and then went down with us to the San Francisco Bay Area to attend Nancy's graduation ceremony. A month or two before Nancy's graduation, there were already five companies intended to recruit her, but she said she wouldn't leave the Bay Area. So she chose a company in San Francisco to work after graduation.

The five of us happily drove to Monterey, a famous tourist destination south of San Francisco. I think back then, this was the first city where Gene and I dated. I remembered it was the local Indian Summer. Because of Monterey's special location, the bay is very deep. There is a Grand Canyon at the bottom of the sea. This moderated the temperatures so there is no hot summer or cold winter. May, June, July and August were often foggy, windy and cold. In the morning it is always 11, 12 degrees Celsius. However, in September and October, the weather is warmer and sunny. Daytime temperature often reaches 25 degrees Celsius. The local autumn is known as "Indian Summer."

I remembered one thing, over ten years ago, it was October 12 (Columbus Day). Gene took me for sightseeing in Monterey. As soon as I saw the sun shining, the blue sea, the blue white clouds, I changed into swimming suit and ran into the cold sea, as the weather was very warm that day. I didn't know the water temperature was always 55 degrees Fahrenheit (equivalent to 12.3 degrees Celsius) no matter how hot it was outside the water. After a few minutes of swimming, I was like a popsicle and inhaled the cool air. I have swum in Houhai, summer palace, canal next to foreign trade institute, Qingshui River in Guizhou, Beidaihe, Qingdao, Dalian, Hawaii, Mexico, but it was never as cold as that time. The sea chilled me to the bone. After swimming in the water for less than ten minutes, I swam back to the beach, only to see a few children playing by the shore. There was no adult in the water. Gene used his camera to catch a shot of my daring to the ocean to swim. When later we moved to Monterey, he still joked with me that "I wanted to see you run into the bay and swim."

Now we were at Monterey Bay again. After seeing Ru Yan and her husband off, I suddenly had an idea: Since Gene is going to retire at the end of the year, and Nancy found a job in San Francisco, Why not finding a teaching job in this beautiful Monterey? I have a master's degree. I am eligible to apply for teaching college. This new idea changed my life.

Chapter 13

A New Life in Monterey

After I told Gene about my idea of looking for a job in Monterey, he was very supportive. We renewed the hotel for two more nights. I started with the local tourist center and asked how many universities there were and where they were. They told me there were two schools to consider. One is Monterey State University(CSUMB) and the other is Monterey Peninsula Community College (MPC). Gene was surprised and asked me, you don't know anyone, where would you start? I said let's go to the personnel offices of the two universities and ask about it. When I asked at the personnel office of the community college, they happened to be recruiting English teachers to "work hourly," that was, to work no more than 20 hours a week, without any benefits, no medical insurance, and no retirement benefits. I thought it was the starting point so I asked for the application form. As for the California State University of Monterey Bay there were no English teachers' position available, but they suggested that I send them my resume. With a glimmer of hope to find a job in Monterey, I drove back to Crescent City with Gene.

About a month after I sent the application form, the Community College Human Resources office informed me that I had been selected by the school to be interviewed and take an exam of English. I drove 350 miles from Crescent City, staying in my daughter's apartment for one night, and then drove 120 miles the next day to be interviewed and took an exam at the English Center in Monterey Community College. There were already three examiners waiting for me: one was the director of the English Center, who seemed very enthusiastic and asked me a few questions. The second was an older English teacher who didn't ask many questions. The third was a young computer expert who asked me mainly what computer software I could use and whether I knew how to use a website. The director told me that their three-person recruiting team would wait until they had my English exam and then select one from people who applied for the job. It took me less than an hour to complete the three page exam paper, most of which were English grammar questions. When I was studying English at Beijing Foreign Trade Institute, one of my strongest subjects was English grammar, so I confidently turned in the papers. The director said I would hear from the college within two weeks.

Sure enough, I quickly received a job offer from Monterey Peninsula Community College. I was informed that the school year would start on Monday, August 21, 2000, but there would be a faculty meeting before the school started, from 1:00 p.m. to 5:00 p.m. on August 18. I needed to attend the faculty meeting for the fall and meet with colleagues. Gene and I were overjoyed that there would be finally a hope to return to San Francisco Bay Area! Although the salary was not high, I said that I could temporarily rent a room in a single family home, cook for myself, and then rent an apartment after the end of the year when Gene planned to join me.

I put an advertisement in the local Monterey newspaper that a female teacher needed to rent a room in a house. I received three replies by phone within a few days. Gene and I decided to drive down and meet the owners. We chose the home of an 82- year-old woman of Hispanic origin on Pebble Beach. I had a very small room with a bathroom. The kitchen and laundry room were shared with the owner.

The rent was $500 per month. We two ladies accepted each other.

Life is a circle. What I want to tell you here in advance is that 16 years later, the house I bought in 2016, the 10,000-square-foot yard, the home of 2700 square feet, is just behind this same old lady's house. Of course she was long gone. I never dreamed that I would buy a house in a wealthy area, and it was right behind the house I rented 16 years ago! Is there such a coincidence in the world? It's incredible. Maybe God sees me struggling with life, and he blessed me? Or could it be that my ancestors have virtue and blessings for their descendants?

Nancy was of course very happy that I found a job in Monterrey. She went to work in San Francisco, which was a two hour drive from Monterey. What excited me even more was that before I moved from Crescent City to Monterey, I was hired by CSUMB to teach English writing . I would teach afternoon classes twice a week for two hours each time. There was no conflict with the morning hours at the English Center of the Community College. In fact, this second job was recommended by Wanda, the director of the English Center of Community Colleges. She told me that the head of the English department at the CSUMB asked her to recommend a teacher who could teach first-year English writing classes. The job was also an hourly contract teacher with no benefits except for salary, no health insurance, and no retirement pay. Wanda felt it might be too tight for me to live in Monterey with one part time job, plus I got a perfect score on my English grammar test. She also had a good impression of me during the interview. So she recommended me. I ow many thanks to her!

The head of the English department at CSUMB (Diana) considered that I lived in Crescent City and it was too far to drive down to Monterey for an interview. She arranged an hour interview on the phone before she decided whether to hire me or not. The phone interview went well. She was satisfied with the answers to questions about how to teach English writing, how to deal with students who are struggling to learn, how to deal with students with different family backgrounds, and so on. On the spot, she announced that she formally hired me as a teacher of writing in the English Department of Monterey State University. Both universities sent me letters of employment and pre-faculty meetings and schedules for the start of the semester.

The faculty meeting at Monterey State University is scheduled for August 16, 17, and 18, Wednesday through Friday. The faculty meeting for Monterey Community College Faculty was scheduled for Friday, August 18, from 1 to 5 p.m. Gene and I were overjoyed! After 11 years, our wish to return to the San Francisco Bay Area finally came true!

I have worked in different organizations in China for 19 years. I deeply felt that we were still dominated by Confucianism and feudalist ideology. The subordinates have to obey the superiors whether it is right or wrong. If you are asked to go to the east, you cannot go to the west; if you are given an apple to eat, you cannot eat a pear. There is no personal will, no freedom of choice. Even wearing clothing, one has to consider his/her age and people around him/her. You can't choose the work you want to do or even choose a spouse! One has to obey the leader and listen to the parents. Otherwise you will become the target of everyone or become a rebel. One has to listen to all the gossip about you. People blame you, and some leaders may not like you. In Chinese we say you have to wear small shoes and suffer from it, but you can't do anything about it. Once you have a bad entry in your file, it will stay with you for your lifetime. It sounds unbelievable, but that is the reality in China.

Working in the United States, it seems that there are not so many rules and regulations as long as you do the work entrusted to you well. No one interferes with your personal life. You can give full play to your abilities. Creativity and ideas that are beneficial to work are always encouraged and supported. You can choose what to wear, where to live, where to work, where you want to go, what kinds of friends you want to make, and say what you want to say. Some people may disagree with my words above. "Is the moon in the United States rounder than in China??" More round or less round, each has its own experience and each has its own vision. What I said is just based on my own experience. There are two sides to everything in the world. There will never be only one side. Choose what you believe. There is no need to argue.

I remember staying in China for nearly half a year when I returned to China to visit my relatives and friends at the age of 52. I had the privilege of meeting a living Buddha. At a meeting there were three Buddhist friends, a sister told me that I might have a disaster at the age of 55. I didn't take it seriously. I was excited to start my new life in Monterey.

Chapter 14

An Awkward Meeting

In 2000, Nancy was studying as an undergraduate student at the University of Berkeley's School of Engineering. She suddenly called me in early January and told me that her dad had lead an education delegation on a tour to the eastern part of the United States. Bingsheng's leader told him that he didn't need to go back with his delegation to China. They gave him a week to spend time with his daughter in the west coast! I was very excited after Nancy's phone call. Bingsheng and I broke up for ten years and now I finally had the opportunity to reunite with the original family of three in the United States! This is because there is always a place in my heart for him and above all he is my daughter's father, my first love, and the husband that I will never forget. I looked forward to meeting and talking to him. Legally we are not husband and wife any longer, but I think we are still a family and we can still be special friends.

I asked Nancy to ask her dad if I could drive down from Crescent City to meet him in the Bay Area. The answer came back, "Let her decide for herself." That was his answer. I felt the chill in my bone and was at a loss what to do. When I talked to a close friend about it many years later, she said, "Wang Bingsheng's answer is right. If he let you come, you are already another man's wife. He might not know whether it is convenient or not; Ifhe asks you not to come to meet him, after all, you were a loving couple, and you have Nancy, why wouldn't he want to see you?" I think she is right. Why am I always so arbitrary and incomprehensible? When I asked Gene whether I should go or not, he said, "You should go down and see Nancy and her father. It will be convenient to have your car to take them around." So with great enthusiasm and expectation, I drove 350 miles heading to Nancy's dormitory. Nancy contacted her father. We planned to go to the airport the next day to pick him up.

When we arrived at S.F. airport, I parked on the side of the road at the exit and asked Nancy to get out of the car to meet her father. After a while, I saw Nancy return by herself. I asked, "What about your father?"

She said, "The Chinese Consulate in San Francisco also sent a Lincoln sedan to pick up him. My dad has asked you to lead the way to my dorm in Berkeley." The man I had been looking forward to meeting for such a long time did not even show his face. I was very disappointed. I failed to understand why he did not let me and my daughter pick him up at the airport, having the consulate people also come to pick him up. If I had known that was the case, why would I have come to the airport? However, I also understand that he is an official of the Ministry of Foreign Affairs and the consulate service comes out of courtesy.

My daughter joked with me when she got in my car, "Wow! They drove a Lincoln limousine while you also drove a Lincoln Town car. Cool! No less than them." When I arrived at the garage of my daughter's dormitory in Berkeley, she opened the fenced door for me with a remote control. As soon as I got in and parked the car, the large fenced door of the garage automatically closed. I stood in the garage, looking out on the street from the iron railing of the fenced gate, not knowing where to get out. I felt like a prisoner. Nancy was busy meeting her father as if she had forgotten my existence. After a while, two drivers from the Chinese Consulate with luggage appeared outside the fenced door with Nancy and her father. It was January. There was no sun on that day, a typical Bay Area day with cloud. It was always cold and gloomy. Bingsheng wore a black tweed coat, a tweed top hat, a pair of black boots, and at a height of 5.90 he looked even taller. He also looked serious and magnificent.

I just ate "two popsicles." The first one: He didn't sit in my car and didn't even see me at the airport. The second one: the four of them were talking and laughing on the road where pedestrians were passing by, but I was trapped in the cold garage inside the fence. I had to smile bitterly and said, "Nancy, you have to let me out!" She realized my embarrassment and said apologetically,"Oh, I'm sorry." She quickly opened the door with the remote control. I felt like a freed prisoner. I walked up the road. For some reason, Bingsheng and I didn't even say hello or shake hands. I walked up to the two drivers and said, "Would you like to come in?" They waved their hands politely and said, "No, we're okay. We have to go back."

Nancy, her father, and I walked into the apartment. After sitting down, it seemed awkward that no one had anything to say, and I didn't know where my excitement had gone. All in all, during that week, every day I drove them out to do some shopping or just walk around. As soon as he got into the car, he sat in the passenger's seat and leaned his head against the window, half-closed his eyes, didn't say a word. When we got back to Nancy's apartment, he sat down on the balcony and smoked one cigarette after another. I made a very simple meal. When eating he and Nancy joked around, but never looked at me once. At night he slept with his daughter in the living room and I slept in Nancy's room. Sometimes I felt too embarrassed to be silent, so I just asked about our old classmates how they were, or how he was doing.

Bingsheng always answered politely and simply. The conversation between the two of us sounded like we were beating around the bush. I felt very distant, and far away from him and it seemed there was a deep ditch between us. I asked him what his impression of the United States was and he said expressionlessly, "Actually, the United States is just so comparing to China, in many ways the U.S. is inferior to China, even more backward than China." Only then did I realize that we were already and indeed two people of two worlds.

I really feel that words of more than half a sentence between the two of us seemed more than enough. I kind of regretted the decision to drive so far to see his icy face. His name is Wang Bingsheng, and his English name is Ice. Did his name really work? After a few days, I hated myself for no self-consciousness. There is Chinese slang to describe my situation: 'Use a hot mouth to kiss that cold ass.' I wanted to drive back right away. My enthusiasm, dreams, and whimsy were all deflated. The unforgiving reality was like a whip whipping my mind, my heart and spirit every day.

I pretended not to see this and coped, until the night before his departure. I couldn't hold back any longer. I was depressed, bitter, bitten, disappointed, and remorseful about making the wrong decision to drive myself down. I felt there was a volcano burning in my heart. I went back to the room where I was sleeping, picked up the phone, and dialed the number of my close friend Rena. I cried as I spoke.

She was an extremely intelligent, considerate, analytical and comforting lady. My daughter realized I had gone and walked into the room, seeing me crying on the phone. She was upset, overwhelmed, and said to me, "What's wrong? What's wrong? Why are you crying?" She has a deep affection for his father. It was a great joy to see her father in the United States. I couldn't bear to let her worry about me anymore; neither did I want to tell her what I had been going through. I didn't believe that she could understand my inner feelings. So I burst into a smile and said, "It's okay, you go and talk to your dad. He'll be leaving tomorrow." Later she relayed her father's words: "Tomorrow the consulate staff will pick him up and take him to the airport, so don't bother to go to the airport."

I didn't know when we would see each other again. I didn't say a word, though I planned to tell him everything in my mind and heart. The enthusiasm, expectation, and excitement that I brought with me were written in a letter, including my pain, regret and disappointment. I put the letter in a big envelope.

The next morning I handed it over to him and asked him to read it on the plane. After he left, I said goodbye to Nancy and drove my Lincoln back to Crescent City. It was strange that it was also cloudy that morning. It did not rain, but the fog in the bay felt as if it were raining lightly. I drove on the Bay Bridge, thinking about my failed journey. My heart seemed carrying a heavy stone. A week ago, I drove down with great excitement but a week later, I left with sadness and disappointment. Uncontrollable tears ran down my face like rain.

How can a couple who were once so loving now seemed even less than strangers?! The hurt I inflicted on him was expressed in the last sentence of the last letter he wrote to me: "This hatred goes on indefinitely " Now he hurt to me so much which made me ask myself if this longing feeling was finally gone! I don't know how many tears I shed that day, as if there were endless springs gushing out my eyes. I drove along 101 North for more than two hours and arrived at Ukiah.

It is a famous Buddhist college. Many Chinese and foreign people come here to visit, chant Buddhist sutras, and even become monks or nuns. I've been here a few times. My tears finally stopped, but my mood was still chaotic. I decided to stay here for an hour or two.

I went into the hall. There were a lot of people chanting a Buddhist sutra that day. I found a seat and sat down reverently. They were reading a Buddhist sutra. Soon everyone stood up and followed a monk around the hall chanting. That was the first time I saw the chanting ceremony like this. I involuntarily followed everyone as they walked in the hall with the bronze statue of Ten Thousand Buddha. I chanted along them. For about half an hour or so, my grievances, my frustrations, my disappointments, and my pain slowly left me.

When I got back in my car, it was about noon. It was also the time when Ice took off from San Francisco airport. I looked at the blue sky with white clouds. I said silently in my heart, Goodbye! As it relieved, I continued to drive north. It would take another five hours to get to Crescent City. There were hardly any vehicles on the road. I looked to my left and stumbled upon white clouds floating in the blue sky. I couldn't resist parking my car on the side of the road and wanted to take a few photos as a memory of this journey home. Yes! Everything is gone by. No more sorrow!

I suddenly noticed a Buddha statue in the middle of the white clouds! It was as if Shakyamuni was sitting there. I couldn't believe my eyes. I looked closely: it was an image of Buddha's statue! I quickly took out my camera and took a few photos. My heart also calmed down. Is it really the Buddha who is manifesting? Shouldn't I let go of human suffering too?

Later, I heard that Buddha statues often appear in the sky above the City of Ten Thousand Buddhas. Now I'm a believer in that for sure.

I firmly believe that day Buddha had shown himself to me to calm me down and enlightened me how to face reality in life.

Chapter 15

Thunderbolt on a Sunny Day

Since I had two jobs waiting for me in Monterey: English Instructor in the English Center at Monterey Peninsula College (MPC), and English Instructor at California State University of Monterey Bay (CSUMB), Gene and I were planning to drive two cars to Monterey on Monday August 14, 2000. We were excited and ready for our new endeavor.

However, on Friday, August 11, 2000, I received a phone call from the surgeon who treated me before. The secretary of his office said that the doctor was going out of town next week and asked me to go to his office that day. I went to his office nervously. In July I felt a hard lump on my left breast. After a biopsy, the doctor said it was a benign tumor and he gave me a surgery to remove the tumor that was two centimeters in diameter. I recovered well. Was there any problem, I wondered?

I walked into his office and saw him holding a piece of paper in his hand and a serious look on his face. He said gently, 'Tm going to tell you not so much a good news. We biopsied the tumor that was taken out, and in two of the 6 slices we found cancer cells. Our conclusion is that you have invasive, malignant breast cancer. I know you've got a new job at Monterrey, but you need surgery as soon as possible... " I didn't hear anything else he said, the news was as deafening as thunder on a sunny day!

"How is this possible?! Isn't God kidding me?"

When I calmed down, I asked him what kind of surgery I would have. He said that to be on the safe side, it was best to have a total left breast removal because of the diameter and nature of the tumor. No more conservative method would be considered.

I started practicing gymnastics at the age of 12, and later learned all kinds of dances, often performing on stage during the holidays. I love beauty, and I love to wear beautiful clothes, how can I lose a breast? (Later, I heard that Chen Xiaoxu, a famous TV star who played Lin Daiyu in the "Dream of the Red Mansion," also had breast cancer. Because she could not bear the shame of losing a breast, she did not use Western medical treatment and chose to enter the Buddhist temple in L.A.. She died within a few years.) Besides, I'm moving to beautiful Monterey next week to start new jobs at two universities, how could I possibly have surgery right away? I could not believe this cruel reality. Sadness, disappointment, helplessness, despair took over my whole body and mind. I put my head on the table and started to cry.

The lady who called me earlier handed me a few napkins, but her sympathetic look couldn't help me. The doctor patiently waited for me to finish crying and said, "If you don't want to stay in the area for surgery, I know a surgeon in Monterey. I can give him a call and arrange for you to see him next week. Whether to stay here for surgery and then rest and give up your new jobs or go to Monterey for surgery and rest there, you can decide for yourself. As for your new job, whether you can get them to keep it for you, I can't say for sure. Well, why don't you go discuss this with your husband over the weekend and call me next Monday with your decision, okay?"

I said, "Aren't you out of town next week?"

"I asked my secretary to tell you that. It was an excuse so I could talk to you in person, I didn't want you to be nervous." What a kind and thoughtful doctor!

I left the doctor's office dazed and don't know how I drove home safely. These were the words in my head: breast cancer, mastectomy. How can a beauty lover like I was bear the shame of losing a breast? A thought of taking my own life suddenly came into my mind. I can take over doze sleeping pills and leave all these behind. If I ended my life, I would not have to suffer, but how would my lovely only daughter suffer? What about Gene who loved me and treated me like a goddess? What about my close relatives and friends? What to do? What to do? What to do? I can put an end to my suffering, but can the pain I inflict on them rest my soul? I can't be so selfish, I have to endure the pain and live! The strength of the Manchu woman's refusal to accept defeat suddenly erupted from my blood. I stood in the courtyard, with no one around, looking at the blue sky, without a trace of clouds, looking at the various fruit trees and lush trees planted by my own hands and Gene, I made up my mind to accept the punishment of fate and accept the test of God. I swallowed back the tears and went back to the room.

I decided to give my good friend who was practicing ballet with me, Linda, a phone call. As soon as she heard it, she said, "Oh, no, no. Too bad." Then she said to me, "I suggest you go to Monterey for surgery. It's an upscale residential area with excellent services in every way. Besides, you may be able to keep your job." I called my eldest cousin, who was the head of the oncology department in Beijing Air Force Hospital. She said don't hesitate to do the surgery and do it as soon as possible. I immediately called my doctor and asked him to help me contact Monterey's doctor. At this critical moment, I had someone to listen to my complaints, comfort me, and help me to decide what to do. How precious! These are my angels.

I already knew what I should do next. When Gene returned from work, I bravely told him the unfortunate news and told him about my decision. He was very surprised and took me in his arms in pain and said, "I will still love you as much as before and I will accompany you to Monterey next week." The love, support and understanding from Gene calmed me down.

The whole weekend was like a dream. I was shedding tears while packing up my clothes. Sometimes I couldn't help but lie on a pile of unfolded clothes crying. I couldn't believe that a "terminal illness" had come to me before I started my new life in Monterey.

My doctor called me on Monday morning and told me that it had been arranged. I would meet with the surgeon in Monterey at ten o'clock on Tuesday morning. He gave me the doctor's name, phone number, and address. On Monday morning, Gene and I each drove a car toward Monterey. The mileage is 420 miles. We arrived in the evening at 4049 El Bosque in Pebble Beach that was my new residence rented a month ago. As I mentioned before after 16 years since I moved to Monterey, the house Daniel and I bought as our home was right across the back yard from the 4049 El Bosque. It is 4138 Crest Road! Talking about life is a circle!

Passing through San Francisco on the way to Monterey, Gene asked me whether I should tell my daughter, Nancy, what happened. I said she had just started her first job after college, I didn't want her to be sad for me and worries about me. I didn't want to affect her mood and decided not to tell her. Gene said what if she would complain afterwards that you didn't tell her about such a big thing in case something happened to you? I said, "If something happens to me, let her always remember what I looked like when I was healthy."

The next day was Tuesday. After examination the doctor decided to give me a mastectomy on Thursday. On Wednesday I went to Monterey State University for teachers' training. I met Director Diana, who hired me on the phone. I also attended meetings for the whole day. I received the schedule of my classes and the list of enrolled students. I told the person in charge that I had an appointment with a doctor the next day and could not participate in the training. She said it was important to see the doctor and there was no need to come for additional training.

On Thursday morning, Gene and I arrived at Monterey Hospital (CHOMP). As soon as we entered the hall, we were both stunned: What kind of hospital is this? It looked like a five-star hotel. There was no taste of 'hospital' at all. The large windows let in bright sunlight, the walls were full of beautiful paintings, the floors were paved with beautiful tiles, and the comfortable sofas were just so inviting. There was also a large pool in the center of the hall, where goldfish swam around in graceful circles. There was a small table next to the pool where you could order a variety of sandwiches, coffee, snacks, etc. My nerves immediately relaxed.

Outside the operating room, we did not wait long before the nurse came out. Gene looked at me affectionately and said, "I'll wait for you to return." I changed my clothes and saw that the doctor who saw me yesterday, whom I hardly recognized, had also changed into his blue-green surgical gown and hat. He said, "We'll give you an anesthesia injection first, When you wake up, everything will be done." He also smiled and asked me, "Are you ready?"

I said, "Isn't it just a piece of meat? Of course! I am ready." Actually, I was only cheering myself up. Hearing my answer to his question in such a dramatic tone of voice prompted he and the nurses to laugh. The tense atmosphere in the room immediately eased. I don't know where I inherited this spirit: In front of big disaster or difficult situation I can tell myself to face it without panic, just concentration on handling the issue.

When I woke up, I only felt that there were thick bandages wrapped around my chest. I had no pain and no odd feelings. When the nurse pushed me out of the operating room, Gene rushed to the side of the gurney. I saw his blue eyes filled with loving sympathy and tears. I smiled and said, "It is over."

This "battle" against cancer has completely changed my outlook on life. I have touched the door of death. What else is there to be afraid of in the world? While losing a breast, I gained a precious spiritual wealth that money can't buy. As for face, fame, money, status, promotion, ups and downs, difficulties, I could care less now. I love everything the Creator has given me more; I love my family and friends more; I love life so much more. The next day after the operation, at 11 a.m. on Friday August 18, 2000, Gene picked me up from the hospital. He said, "Let's go home." I put the vial which carried the liquid flowing from my body into it into my left trouser pocket, put on my coat, and said, "Drive me to the English Center at Monterey Peninsula College." He was shocked, "What? Are you going to the faculty meeting?" I said, "Yes!"

He looked at me and heard my resolute voice. He had no choice but kept saying, "I cannot believe it. I cannot believe it." I endured the pain and slowly walked into the English center located in MPC library. Except for the three teachers who interviewed me in July, the other faculty members, almost a dozen of them, met me for the first time. Director Wanda enthusiastically introduced me to everyone. They are all English teachers. I felt that there was a natural connection with them. Later, I became good friends with them for many years. By five o'clock in the afternoon, Gene was already waiting outside the library. When I got into the car, he had tears in his eyes and said movingly, "You made it!"

Gene stayed with me for two weeks, picking me up and dropping me off from work every day. But he had to go back to Crescent City to do what he needed to do. I was able to drive my car. As for cancer surgery, I never mentioned it to any of my colleagues or students. The vial of liquid was always hidden in my left trouser pocket. Every hour or so I went to the bathroom to pour out the oozing liquid from my body. Fortunately my longest working hours were only four hours. After two weeks the vial will no longer be needed. In retrospect, I don't know how I spent those days. My cognitive abilities seem to have been sublimated by several steps. I have learned that human endurance and perseverance are infinite. It can work wonders. Since then, I have become even bolder than before. It seems that I am not afraid of anything. Nothing is difficult for me. There is no such thing as a road that goes to nowhere. There will be a road before the car reaches the foot hill. Those who have a will succeed in everything. I have personally experienced this.

However, greater trials and embarrassments came into my life. Under the persuasion of the doctor and the head nurse, twenty-eight days after the operation, I began chemotherapy. Once every three weeks, four chemotherapy treatments in total. In order not to affect my work, I scheduled the chemo on Friday afternoons. Three large tubes of liquid were transfused into my veins and it took more than two hours. When I think about it now, I can't believe how I survived all those hardships.

It wasn't painful or too much to feel when I was in infusion, but it was boring and lonely to lie there for more than two hours.

I couldn't watch the TV when the nurse turned it on for me. What tormented and embarrassed me was that after the infusion, on a few occasions, I wet my pants without even noticing it. Back in the room I rented, I vomited, and had no appetite at all. It's like a dragon has been sucked out of its muscles and bones. There was no energy left in me. When I wanted to sleep lying on the bed, but I could not sleep. I didn't tell any of my colleagues or students about my cancer and chemotherapy. In this way, I treated myself as a "healthy person." At school, I acted as a normal teacher, going to class on time, leaving work on time, grading homework. Sometimes my eyes refused to stay open. I had to use cold water to rinse, rub it with my hands, and force myself to finish grading homework. I had to write comments on their papers and explain to the students. Those days and nights of torture were so terribly painful. It is not like I was fighting with disease, but like I was fighting with Fate, fighting with the devil who wanted to devour my will to live. I made up my mind to fight to the end and spell out a way of my life!

The most terrible experience was two weeks after chemotherapy. As the doctor had warned me, my hair was going to fall out. Chemotherapy began on September 15, 2000; on September 30, 2000, I happened to be driving to Sacramento State University, California's capital, for an academic conference. The main reason I went to the meeting was so that I could pass by my daughter's dormitory in Berkeley for the night to see her. I could also tell her about my surgery, I think when she sees me in person and I am still alive she wouldn't worry too much.

When I started to tell her that her mom's health had run into big trouble, her hands clenched into fists; she started to get nervous trembling. She said, "Please tell me quickly." I said calmly, 'Tm okay now, but don't be so nervous. I was diagnosed with breast cancer before moving to Monterey and had surgery on August 17th. It's all in the past."

She couldn't believe her ears. "Now is it really over?" she asked. "There's no danger anymore?"

I said, "Look, I'm right in front of you. It is over. I didn't tell you before, because I was afraid of scaring you."

Relieved, she said, "That's fine." The hardest part of life is telling your loved ones you have cancer. I am proud that I arranged this matter quietly and smoothly to clear this hurdle with my daughter.

After we finished dinner, when I was taking a shower and washing my hair, suddenly a large amount of hair came off my scalp. I was so frightened that I turned off the faucet immediately. I knew that hair loss had started as scheduled. I quickly dried my hair, did not dare to tell my daughter, quietly cleaned up the hair in the bathtub, wrapped it in papers and threw it into the garbage can. Early the next morning, I drove to Sacramento State University where I finished the conference and then returned to a very old high-end hotel in downtown Sacramento reserved by the school for me. When I was taking a shower before going to bed, an even more terrible thing happened.

As soon as I combed my hair, oh my God, it was as if someone pulled my whole scalp off. As soon as my hand touched my hair, a large handful of hair fell out, which frightened me, and before long, the whole bathtub was full of hair falling off my head. After turning off the water , I sat there and couldn't believe my eyes. How could it be that I had so much hair which densely covered the bottom of the tub! What if it really blocked the sewers of this hotel? Fortunately, I turned off the faucet on time and blocked the hair with my hands. I picked up the hair on the bottom of the bathtub with both hands, then I wrapped a pile of hair in into a few napkins and put them in the trash can. Only then did I have time, put on my clothes, but dared not to look myself in the mirror.

However, I did. My God! The black hair on my skull had fallen off a big a quantity. My skull appeared bald in several places. How do I go back to school to see people! Fortunately, no one at the Sacramento State University knew me. On my way back I didn't go to see my daughter after the meeting. I drove straight back to Monterey, found a shop selling wigs in Seaside and bought a wig. October is called Indian Summer in California, as previously described: three months of summer in Monterey, June, July and August, it is mostly foggy, and the temperature can be as low as 50 (F)12 Degrees (C) The sun begins to shine brightly after September, and the temperature can reach 80 (F) 25 (C). Putting on the wig was unbearable. My scalp was itchy and I felt panic, so I thought of a way to wrap my head with a silk scarf. Every day I had a different beautiful scarf. When I got home, I finally became myself, feeling awful, miserable and terrible, but safe.

I now couldn't believe that I didn't cry in those horrible days. On the contrary I gritted my teeth, going to face my co-workers and students every day without telling them what I had been suffering. I even kept going to my ballet class while wearing a wig. I had to hold onto it when I did back stretching for fear it might fall off and scare the whole class. I went swimming with my right arm paddling the water. I did not stop my tennis lesson on Friday either. I just lived life as it came, normally. I was determined to fight and win this battle.

This big tree in Pebble Beach near the 18-hole located near the Lodge witnessed the emotions I had after surgery and

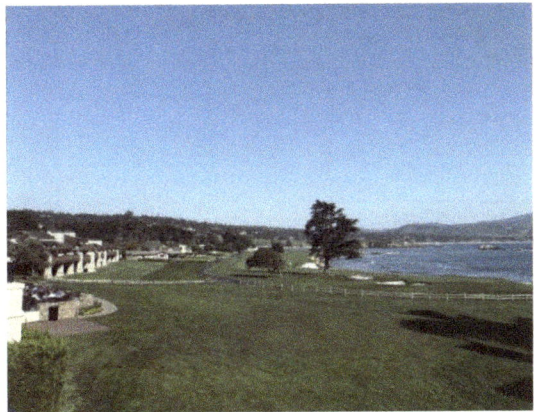

chemotherapy in the summer of 2000. Every weekend I drove from the room I rented in El Bosque of Pebble Beach to come here to do qigong. (Gene hadn't moved to Monterey yet).

From the tree I could look out on the golf course and the Lodge and encouraged myself not to feel sad or give up because life is beautiful. I firmly believe where there is a will there is a way.

On April 6, 2022, Sara, Daniel's sister, accompanied me to this corner reminiscing the most difficult time in my life: 22 years ago, every weekend I came here to ease my loneliness, the pain, and the torment of the loss of my left breast and the side effects of terrible chemotherapy. Looking at the world's most famous scenery, the sky without a trace of cloud and the blue sea, I absorbed the energy given to me by the infinite universe. Now no words can express the happiness in my mind! How could I not love life and the world?

A semester later, in January 2001, I was hired to teach Tai Chi

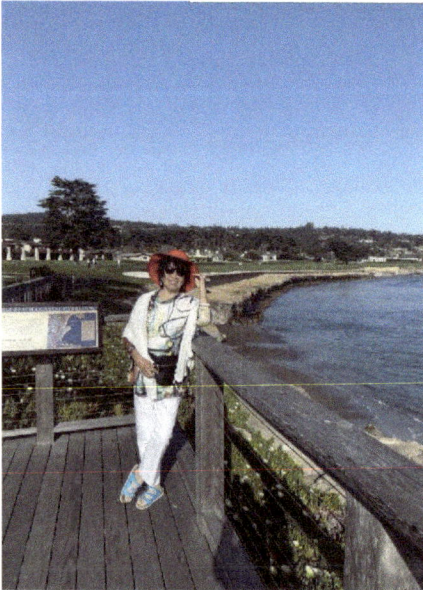

every Saturday morning at Monterey Community College. In the first Tai Chi class, when I told everyone how I used Qigong and Tai Chi to fight against cancer. I saw a few colleagues from the English Center who supported me to sign up for the Tai Chi class, covering their mouths with their hands and widening their eyes. We spent more than three months together from August to mid-December, and I couldn't bear to tell them that I had breast cancer and went to work with a disease. Now they all knew the truth, after class, they all came up to me and hugged me. I was strong for a few months, but then I couldn't hold back my tears any longer. We were all crying. One of them said, "I see you wear all kinds of scarves, because you always wear beautifully, I thought it was one of your outfits. I've doubted whether you're going through chemotherapy, but I'm embarrassed to ask you. You should have told us earlier, and we can help you. At least we can share with you your sorrow."

What great colleagues!

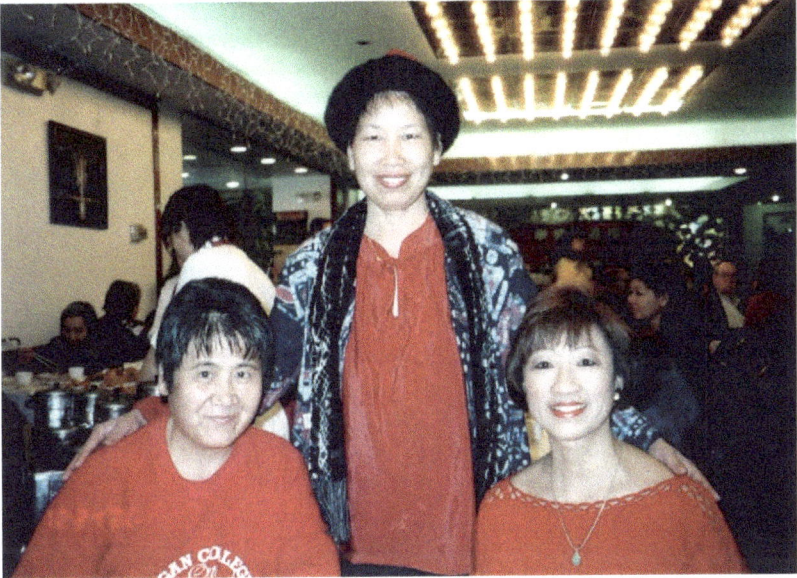

My friend Susie came to see me and we ate hot pot with Rena.

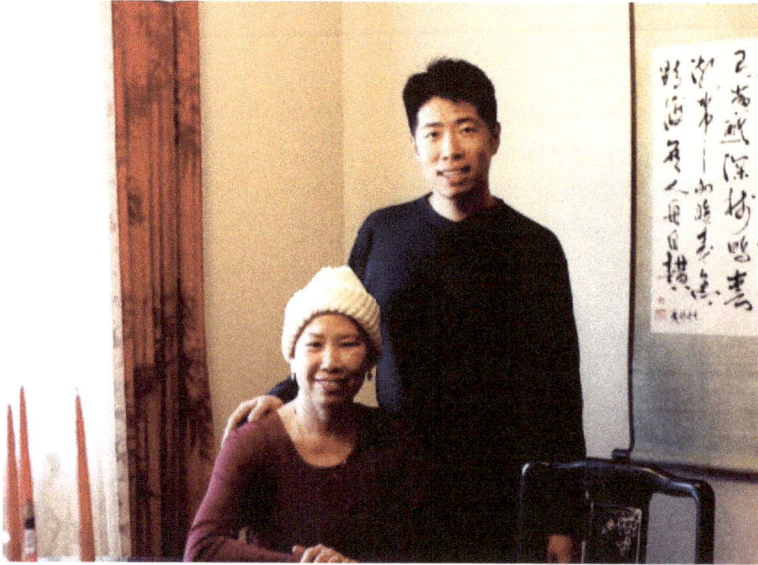

Chen Yue, the eldest son of my cousin came to Monterey to visit me while I went through the second round of Chemo

In October 2000, Gene also retired from his job in Crescent City Senior Center in northern California and moved to Monterey. Because the Delmont County Senior Center where he worked was an nonprofit organization with no benefits, I had to look for a full-time job with full health insurance and a pension. As the saying goes, when one door in your life closes, another door is open to you. One day, one of my Tai Chi students said to me, "You should go to the Defense Language Institute in Monterey Fortress to teach Chinese, which is a government department with good health insurance and retirement benefits." I said to Gene that I wanted to go there to have a look. He said,it's an army fortress, whom are you going to find. I said, "let's go and ask where the personnel office is."

To put the long story short, June 25, 2001, I started working full-time in DLI (The Defense Language Institute) under the U.S. Army of D.O.D (Department of Defense) at the Presidio of Monterey in California, USA teaching Chinese. The students were selected from among U.S. Army, Navy, and Air Force officers and soldiers to serve in the military with certain language skills. Most of them are around twenty years old, full of vitality and enthusiasm. As soon as I entered the classroom and saw their glowing eyes and eagerness to learn, I forgot that I was a cancer patient who had just recovered. I not only taught them Chinese pronunciation, grammar and various sentence patterns, but also introduced Chinese culture, history, and customs in combination with the language. I also use various lively activities to kead them into dialogue, such as role-playing. When I saw that the students were sleepy and tired, I also spent three or two minutes leading them to do a few Tai Chi movements. Soon I became a favorite teacher for my students. As soon as several students saw me approaching the classroom, they sat up straight, smiles on their faces, and some simply said, "Ah, my favorite teacher Li is here." Teaching in such an atmosphere, I was happy every day. I also continued to play ping-pong, tennis, swimming, ballet lessons, and taught Tai Chi on weekends. My cancer doctor, Dr. Jerome Rubin, supported all my activities and supported me in taking some Chinese herbs to help get rid of the side effect of chemo. He was very happy for my rapid recovery and extraordinary energy. He told me he often used me as an example to inspire other patients.

One February night in 2002, next to the ping-pong table, I was smashing a forehand ball when I suddenly felt a lower back pain. I thought maybe I put too much power to hit the ping pong ball. I went to visit Dr. Howard, a local cervical spine specialist, who examined me and asked me to go to a physiotherapy center in Carmel. After two or three months of physiotherapy twice a week, my back pain didn't get any better. The young man who gave me the physiotherapy reported to Dr. Howard that I was not getting better. Dr. Howard asked me to come to his office and took a few large lumbar spine X-ray for me. After a while he walked in and he looked at me disappointedly and said, "No wonder your back pain can't be cured! Look, there's a hole in the middle of the fifth section of your lumbar spine!" (I kept that X ray film for more than a decade and tossed it away before I went to Italy.) I sat there dumbfounded and listened to him saying, 'Tm just a cervical and spine specialist. I think there might be three reasons for this hole: one is osteoporosis, but the disease is not common in the Asian population; the second is that as you said, you twisted your waist when playing, but it is unlikely; and the third reason might be that your breast cancer has metastasized there, and the cancer cells have eaten the bones. But I'm not a cancer expert. You'd better go back to your cancer doctor and check it out."

I called Dr. Rubin with a nervous heart. He asked me to come to his office the next morning. After seeing the X-ray film from Dr. Howard,, he arranged for me to go to CHOMP to have a scan at 7 p.m. on the same day. The next day, I went to his clinic to see the results.

I walked into his office with a horrible feeling of apprehension. Within a few minutes, Dr. Rubin walked in. Looking at his gloomy face, I had a hunch that something was not good-it must be the third case! Sure enough, he whispered, "It's bad news. Your breast cancer has metastasized to 7 parts of your bones in your body." What? Another thunderbolt hit me! I didn't believe my ears, and asked, "How can it be that the cancer has metastasized and not something else?" He explained slowly, "The white liquid you swallowed before the scan yesterday reached your whole body in a few seconds. Wherever there are cancer cells, it will appear obviously white. On your body, we found 7..." Before I could finish listening to his explanation, my tears couldn't help but welled out. After I finished sobbing, he said to me in a comforting tone, "Although this is bad news, what puzzled me and also a good news is your internal organs have not been invaded by cancer cells. In ordinary cases, when cancer cells have attacked 7 places of the bone in your body it should also attack some internal organs, but your lungs, liver, kidneys, and heart are very clean, without a trace of cancer cells. I can't explain this phenomenon. Maybe it has something to do with you practicing Qigong and teaching Tai Chi. The good news is that we can concentrate on dealing only with problems in your bones. I don't have to worry about other organs. As for the hole that was eaten by cancer, it may need to be operated on in the future to punch medical cement into it, but that is later. What we're going to treat is cancer cells that have metastasized to the bones."

"In what way?" I asked. He said, "You're going through a course of chemotherapy. Once every three weeks, for a total of four times.

"Will I lose my hair like last time?" "Sorry, but yes." "Why, is my cancer metastasizing?"

He said, "You had the most malignant kind of invasive breast tumor, which is easily metastasized."

Starting from mid-June 2002, I started another round of chemotherapy treatments again. This time the reaction was even more severe than the first round. I could not eat anything just like the dragon was cramped and weakened. After work, I lay on the couch and lingered. My friend Susie Wang, who just moved to Monterey to live in my house temporarily tried her best to make various meals to persuade me to eat a little. She used to own a restaurant, is a good cook, and her cooking has a full range of colors and flavors. But my sense of taste was killed by the chemotherapy. I didn't have any appetite, and even if raw salt was put on my tongue, it had no taste. Susie has taken care of many elderly people and is very experienced. Seeing my appearance, she quietly and sadly told Gene, "It seems that Lydia is already a terminal patient, you should be prepared for the aftermath." Gene later told me that his answer was, "No, Lydia will not die. She will survive!" After listening to him, I was not only very touched but also encouraged, because Gene was so positive about me, and so positive about my prospects.

I already had the experience of losing my hair earlier. This time I was ready. On the fifteenth day of chemotherapy, as soon as my hair started to fall out, I asked Gene to shave all my hair off. I didn't want to experience the terrible feeling oflosing hair: the whole scalp was like being peeled off by someone else. I took off my headscarf in the office when it was hot. The feeling of the humiliation of being bald was still there, but the skin of my face seemed to be a little thicker. Teacher Wei, an American teacher in the same office, said to me half-jokingly, "Lydia, I wouldn't have known the shape of your head is so perfect when you have hair." That kind of loving, comforting, warm words, moved me deeply. Later, Teacher Wei also asked me and his wife, a professional singer, to perform Chinese folk songs on the local radio station.

My desire to survive this time seemed stronger than the first time. The confidence to fight cancer seemed to be more abundant. I also didn't tell my students. But a female student whose sister had undergone chemotherapy suddenly asked me in class, "Teacher Li, why did you start chemotherapy again?" I was not mentally prepared at all, hesitated, and honestly I said, "because my breast cancer metastasized to my bones." The class was silent. I reassured them that after four rounds of chemotherapy, I would be fine.

When I came home from lunch at noon and came back to my office, I saw a vase on my desk with a beautiful bouquet of flowers and a greeting card on the table with words of encouragement from students signed in Chinese. I don't know whether I was sad or moved, but tears streamed down my face. In the afternoon, the head of the department called me into her office and said to me, "if you need a leave of absence or any help, we will do our best. You can also take time off and rest at home."

I didn't take sick leave. I thought instead of being afflicted by chemotherapy at home and moaning in pain, I would rather think of myself as a normal person who could do whatever I wanted. I'm going to test my God: Let's see ifI'm tough, or you're tough! It isn't a big deal to die, I thought. IfI'm not afraid of death, what else can you do with me? I went to ballet classes with wigs, Chinese lessons with my headscarves, Tai Chi classes with my bald head, and performed at various occasions with beautiful scarves. My life seemed to be unaffected, and I still actively participated in various activities. Only inside of me I did know what it was really like, but the mental willpower triumphed over the physical pain. I was not afraid; I was not depressed; I was not complaining; I was not disappointed. I wanted to live, not only for myself, but also for my family, my students and friends. I love this wonderful world. I am proud, and proud of my strength. (You see, Gene was correct about me. I'm a survivor!)

My eldest sister's second son was as close as a son to me, and I was like his mother. When he heard that my cancer had metastasized, he sent me Chinese Ganoderma lucidum spores (later renamed Shuang Ling Gu Ben San) from Tianjin despite the high price. After eating for a month, I started to have an appetite. By the end of 2002, the tumor indicators gradually returned to normal. Instead of dying, I survived healthily. Every morning between classes, I do Tai Chi exercise in the corridor outside the classroom. Some teachers and students also do it together with me. Many photographs and videos of various occasions in that year recorded that unforgettable historical period.

My story was published in newspapers and magazines and

encouraged many others.

I thank everyone who prayed, encouraged, and helped me to survive this disaster. I am back to my happy and meaningful life again. I will give my love, care, strength and energy to this world.

Chapter 16

My Daughter Started a Family

In 2005, I returned to Beijing to meet with Bingsheng, Nancy's to be in-laws including Nancy and her fiance, Chi. We six people discussed the wedding of our daughter and son in a very fancy seafood restaurant. In May of that year, my son-in law, Chen Chi held a grand wedding ceremony attended by 150 people in the Beijing Jun Wang Mansion (Palace of Prince Jun). At my daughter's wedding, looking at the hall full of dignitaries, relatives and friends, and the joyful atmosphere, I couldn't help but recall how the two met each other. Nancy is a very simple girl. Her heart was like her smooth and delicate skin, white and clear, jade-like and transparent.

When she was in high school in Crescent City, Nancy was the top student of the school and was the President of the International Student Club, the main player of the varsity tennis team, and the most awarded No. 1 speaker of the speech and debate team. A boy asked her out to lunch. Nancy asked me if she could go, I refused absolutely. I treated her just like how my father treated me- no way could she be alone with male classmates. Nancy was not happy with me. But she did what I asked. When Nancy studied at Berkeley, in a conversation with Gene, Nancy said, "I am grateful to my mom. Some of my high school classmates fell in love and some became pregnant before marriage. Some had children and had to drop out of school."

In 2002, the U.S. economy slumped, and many online .COM companies closed down. Nancy returned to Beijing to work in the office of the World Bank. Chen Chi also returned to Beijing due to the closure of his company. His father, and Nancy's cousin Xiao-Hong, worked in a same office. When they were chatting, Mr. Chen learned that Xiao-Hong's cousin, Nancy, did not have a boyfriend, Mr. Chen said that my son and your cousin had returned from the United States, why not let them meet.

"But can I see her first?" This was what Mr. Chen later told me when he came to visit me in the United States. Mr. Chen told me, "I liked your daughter as soon as I saw her. Nancy is not only beautiful and generous, with superior skin, but also has a beautiful demeanor. Now many girls are knowledgeable and have higher degrees. But none of them are as elegant and classic as your daughter."

"So I went home and told my son that I had met Xiao-hong's cousin, Nancy. By then my son hadn't seen Nancy yet, but I was in charge. I told Chen Chi that he must meet her". "You can't let such a wonderful girl marry into someone else's house. She has to be a daughter-in-law to our family." Mr. Chen told me very proudly.

When I heard all these nice comments and thought of Mr. Chen, I didn't expect him to be so frank. I feel so proud of my daughter. I'm glad he chose the daughter-in-law at first glance. After Chen Chi saw Nancy, he started to work on it. Later, Chi told me, "The first time I invited your daughter to dinner, I spent 1500 yuan. She was truly excellent. I decided she should be the mother of my future children."

On Nancy's 24th birthday, Chen Chi ordered 99 red roses and sent them to the World Bank office in Beijing where Nancy was working. When the front desk receptionist announced that Nancy please come to go to the front desk to pick up flowers, everyone in the whole building knew Nancy had a boyfriend who sent big bouquet of roses to the front desk. A colleague also took a photo on the scene. Nancy's photo of struggling to hold 99 roses has remained in my album. Later, when Chen Chi chatted with me to recall the scene, I said, "You are so smart. You have only known each other for two months, but you took that action, which is equivalent to announce to everyone that no one should date Nancy." Chen Chi smiled and replied, "Yes, that's what I meant back then!"

Chi and Nancy both returned to the United States in 2002. The following story is also what Chen Chi told me. Chen Chi was living in Connecticut at the time, while Nancy lived in Emeryville, San Francisco Bay Area, California. In order to be closer to Nancy, Chen Chi found one of his master's classmates, also lived and worked in Emeryville, California. Chi rented one room from his classmate. In this way he could see Nancy easily. His efforts paid off. Looking at this pair of talented lovers get married, how could I not be happy.

One year later they had a son, Aaron, who is now 18, going to George Washington University in August. Five years later a daughter, Audrey was born, who is 12 this year. Those two beautiful and gifted grandchildren have become the source of my pride and joy.

2005 was an auspicious year. I went to Shanghai to watch the National Peking Opera performances. I saw almost all the famous characters of Peking Opera. After attending my daughter's wedding in Beijing, I was invited to the U.S. Embassy in China for lunch with Ambassador Randt and his wife Sarah and their three children. Mr. Randt and I worked for a few years in the Commercial Section of the U.S. Embassy in Beijing (in the Jianguo Hotel) when he was the first secretary of the Commercial Department of the U.S. Embassy in Beijing. I was the chief translator in the Commercial Section of U.S. Embassy stationed in Beijing. We worked well together; worked very productively, and I have had friendly contact with his family since then. A few years later I went to the United States, and Mr. Randt was appointed U.S. Ambassador to China. On Veteran's Day 2006, Gene and I took my friend's daughter, Rebecca Jackson (a Julia School of Music graduate) to the U.S. Embassy in Beijing to perform her violin with my solo singing of Chinese folk songs for the Ambassador and his guests. These were unforgettable moments. In 2005 my life was full of sunshine!

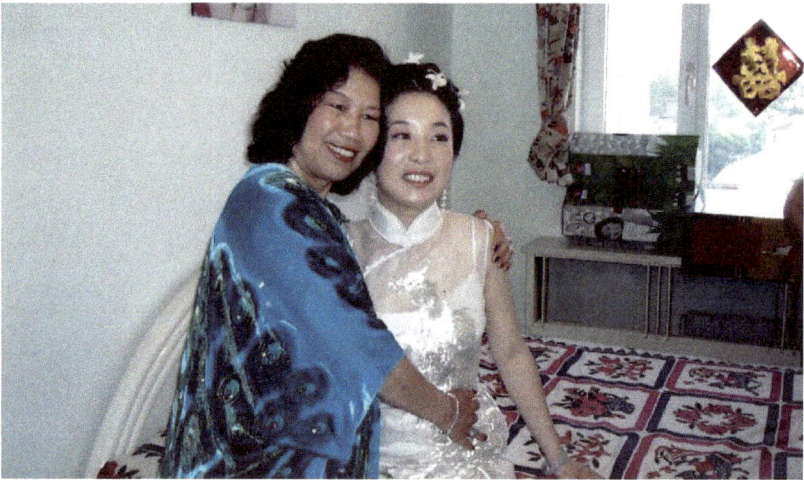

My daughter is getting married!

Chapter 17

My Third Husband Daniel Dieli

It never occurred to me that I would leave Gene. He was such a righteous gentleman. I am an idealist who acts according to feelings, not by mind. It can also be said that I am a woman who is controlled by her own emotions. In many cases, it is life that chooses me, not me who chooses life. Plus our universe is vast, each of us is so small, how much can I control?

Let me begin to write about my third gentleman, my husband, Daniel Dieli. Daniel is 5 feet 8.5 inches tall. After years of martial arts study, and military training, his body is straight and very strong. His hair was wavy. Underneath his glasses were a pair of blue eyes that were always thinking and exploring. He is a typical Italian man with a high bridge nose and a very well shaped small mouth. When he is in a good mood, he is very polite to people. He likes to talk and laugh, is very humorous, responsive, and talented in telling vivid stories.

Sometimes he uses a posture with his right leg and his right hand being pulled down, in standard Beijing dialect, "Your highness Lao Fu Ye. (Empress Zi Ci's nick name) What can I do for you?" I joked back on the spot, "Comb my hair." (Do you believe it, when we were on the streets of Beijing, and when he saw that my hair was messy, he took out a comb from his pocket and brushed my hair on the spot causing my niece who accompanied us to cover her mouth and laugh). The joking conversation between the two of us made everyone laugh. Once, he performed again and when I said, "Bring me a cup of tea," he suddenly said in an authentic, Chinese tone, "Sorry I am busy!" It caught me off guard. "What's wrong with you today? Don't you dare to rebel?" We made everyone laugh. I was wondering where he learned that line. The answer turned out that one ofby my good friends Wang Jing taught him not to obey the empress dowager anymore. However, when he was not happy, he lowered his head, and his face looked like dark clouds. For a long time you could not get a word out of his mouth.

Daniel is very simple, loyal and reliable, absolutely trustworthy, and a good person. He graduated with BA in music education from the Crane School of Music at Suny Potsdam majoring in trumpet and tuba. After graduation, he joined the U.S. Army Military Band, and he had been to the opening and closing ceremonies of the Olympic Games held in various countries. Working in the military band as a tuba player, he was went to South Korea three times. He also played for U.S. military celebrations many times. He learned martial arts from Chinese, Korean, Vietnamese and Japanese, and he studied martial arts from an early age. He also enthusiastically studied Buddhism, reading many books on the subject. He has his own views on politics, the economy, culture, geography and history of all countries around the world. By this time, we had been married for 14 years. His love for me was always so sincere, persistent and profound. Whatever I say, he listened in the ear, remembered in the heart, and took actions right away. Even if he was tired and had different ideas, he still did what I asked. His love for me is as hot as the sun, as if it can melt me. His love towards everyone in my extended family was also from the bottom of his heart, without any reservation. It was so sincere and touching. I often feel that he is water, I am a fish in that water. He is the sea where I can swim. It is incredible to meet him, I already had two husbands who loved me. How lucky I was to have such a third husband?

Now let me tell you how we met. As soon as he moved to the Presidio of Monterey as the manager of the legal office, he began to ask if there were any local teachers who taught Tai Chi. Because he loved Chinese martial arts since he was a child and had studied with Vietnamese martial arts masters in high school in New York State, with South Korean, Japanese and Chinese martial arts masters in San Francisco, with American martial arts masters in Virginia, and so on. All in all, his greatest hobby was oriental martial arts. A Thai-American who works in the computer office told him, "Lily of the Chinese Department (he didn't know my English name was Lydia) taught Tai Chi." Daniel found my office, and I was not there. The fourth time we met, he said he wanted to learn Tai Chi with me one-on-one. I was very surprised. How could such a strong middle-aged man treat me as a martial teacher? Moreover, I am not a Tai Chi master. I just like martial arts and participated in martial arts classes in high school to learn some skills from Tai Chi masters.

Since I came to the U.S. I practiced Tai Chi to eliminate myfrustration and loneliness in difficult situations. I had also performed in different places and taught 24 styles of Tai Chi. Now teaching Tai Chi at a community college on weekends was also a hobby. I told him that I wasn't a martial arts master and it was just my hobby. I told him that I didn't have time to teach individual students. Ifhe wants to learn Tai Chi Style 24 or Style 32 Tai Chi Sword, he may go to the community college to enroll in my class when the spring started. Daniel asked if he could come to my office before community college started. I saw that he was so eager, so I said okay. It was the fall of 2002.

He told people many times of his first meeting with me, "When I found Lydia, she was wearing a hat because it was Indian Summer in Monterey, California. The weather was very hot. She suddenly took off her hat and smiled and said, 'I'm a nun.' I saw she had no hair. My heart trembled: she must going through chemotherapy! Because my second elder sister had breast cancer, went through chemo, and died that year. However, I was struck by Lydia's open-mindedness and optimism. I knew the pain of chemotherapy, but she ignored her own suffering and was afraid that I would be embarrassed and joked with me. What a strong woman! I thought to myself, I can't learn Tai Chi from her. She will definitely die. But somehow she was like a magnet, irresistibly attracting me. I just started working as the manager of the legal office I was not familiar with the environment, so I was confused every day. I had no one to ask for advice. I was nervous and anxious.

I ran to Lydia's office and asked her about Tai Chi movements. She stood in the hallway in front of the classroom, pointed at Monterey Bay and said, "You see, we can see the blue sea, the emerald pine trees, how lucky to work in such an environment!" I was shocked again: she was terminally ill, facing death, undergoing unbearable chemotherapy. She should have no smile. The chemo was very painful and she should have a sad face, but she was still so lively and cheerful and saw the beautiful things in life. I am a man as healthy as a cow complaining about the world, far inferior to her "

Daniel was inspired by my spirit. Later he went to Monterey Community College (MPC) to enroll in my Tai Chi class. The Tai Chi class I taught at a community college every Saturday morning ranges from a dozen people to thirty or forty people each semester. A dozen of them signed up every semester. They were very positive about my teaching methods and personality. A few of them had formed a small group and became my followers. Every Saturday, classes didn't seem to be enough, so I added a free Tai Chi exercise. Every Sunday morning we gathered on the balcony outside the City Hall or on the beach in Carmel to practice the 24 styles of Tai Chi, Qigong, and Tai Chi Sword that I taught them in class. Then we went to a Chinese restaurant for lunch together.

During the holidays, Gene and I invited everyone to come to my house for a party. The students celebrated my birthday which later developed into celebrating each student's birthday at a different restaurant. What touched me the most was that, when I was going through the second round of chemotherapy because my of breast cancer metastasis to my bones, they organized a party to wish me a speedy recovery. Daniel was one of them. I also took them to Tai Chi and Tai Chi Sword performances on various occasions. We were like one big family. Daniel has great respect for me and Gene. He often talked to Gene about the frustration in his work. Gene explained to him, "Your pressure comes down from above because you work for a military organization. There is no choice but obey the orders. There is only strict discipline that cannot be flexible. Just imagine how your supervisors feel; how many orders they have to obey every day from above; how much pressure they have on their shoulders. So the pressure falls upon you." Once Daniel said, " Can you two adopt me?" He seemed so simple and native. We all laughed.

Every time I walked home to eat lunch around noon, passing by his office, he often came out and said, " Can I walk with you to the gate?" During those 5 to 6 minutes' walking, he talked to me about the troubles in his family, his mother's illness, his father's anxiety, his girlfriend's hot temper, and so on. I helped him analyze things and comforted him like a big sister. A few years passed. He was like my little brother!

At that time, our teachers were using computers, and it was

difficult to move the heavy computer with CPU to another office. In addition to filling out work order forms to move the computer and peripherals, one also had to wait for the school technicians to start the computer output. Sometimes it took two or three days before you could use your own computer again. I was temporarily transferred from one team to another very often, because the Dean of the Asian School said, "I don't worry about any shortage of teachers, because I can send Lydia there. She can get along with anyone, the students like her and she works seriously and very responsibly " What else can I say? However, the frequent temporary transfers caused me a lot of inconvenience.

Daniel was so proficient at computers. As soon as I called him for help, he moved the computers to my new office the same day and installed them in less than an hour. Many of the teachers at our school didn't know who Daniel was, but the rumor that "Lydia's Tai Chi student is very loyal to her and is always on call" had been spread about.

Monterey didn't even have a Chinese store, not to mention Chinese artistic performances. There was no internet then. If you want to buy some Chinese groceries, watch Chinese programs, you had to go to the San Francisco Bay Area. I am addicted to Chinese culture. Whenever there were any performances from China, for example, "Yunnan Song and Dance Troupe," Suzhou opera "Peony Pavilion," the Central Orchestra, ballet, "Big Red Lantern Hangs High," the dance drama "Mei Lifang," the play "Sai Jinhua," etc., I would find a few friends to go with. My co workers could drive from home to school every day, but there were very few teachers who could drive out of Monterey because most of us didn't grow up with private cars and few learned to drive after arriving in America. It took at least two hours one way from Monterey to the Bay Area. Every time I asked Daniel if he wanted to go, he always said, "I don't have a social life, I'm willing to go, and I can help you drive back."

After my Tai Chi class on Saturday, I drove my Lincoln sedan, which could hold 6 people, to see performances in the Bay area. Along the way, we talked, joked, and laughed. We passed by Ranch 99 Chinese store to buy groceries before the show and then ate a big meal at a Chinese restaurant before coming back. We all had good times. Daniel always helped me to drive back. Gene was at home enjoying watching his TV and working on his paintings.

In those years, I was fascinated by Peking Opera and participated in Peking Opera clubs in San Francisco Bay Area. When there was a performance, Gene couldn't stand the loud gong and drum beats of Peking Opera. Nor could he stand the high peach voices of the sound. It was also too hard for him to be out town for a few hours, so I asked Daniel to come with me. He became my driver. Our relationship was harmonious and natural. I felt like I was his mom, sister, and of course a teacher. As for what he thought, whether you believe it or not, I never thought about it or didn't ask. Gene and I treated him like a loyal student and little brother, and we were grateful for his help.

Here I would like to add a few words: After my cancer metastasized in 2002, I defeated the cancer and recovered my health due to 1) Ganoderma lucidum herb sent from China by my second nephew Tian Wenshu, 2) the love of my students, 3) the prayers and support of friends and colleagues, 4) the love of Gene, and 5) the company of Daniel, I will never forget these wonderful people. The last but not the least, my passion for life and the desire to live. My Manchu blood made me a tough girl and a fighting woman. I will never give up. I firmly believe the power of one's will can overcome any fear and defeat the enemies in ourselves.

A few years later, two of my Tai Chi students separately

mentioned Daniel's complicated feelings towards me. He was so puzzled and confused, so he confided in two ladies whom he trusted, saying that he had been deeply in love with me for a long time. The two ladies were also my Tai Chi students. The advice they gave him was to encourage him to talk to me openly and honestly. One lady said, Lydia will not get mad at you. As soon as inner thoughts were spoken out, it would be clear and easy to handle. Another lady said that you two were really a complementary couple, but it is a pity that she has a husband who loves her so much, so just forget about it. Just keep the friendship.

Later I learned that Daniel had rejected their advice and continued to have secret feelings for me. He also told them, "Lydia holds high prestige in our community. Many people know and like her. I cannot ruin her reputation because of my feelings. My love for her is to protect her, to help her and not to let her know." The Tai Chi class I taught was from 9 a.m. to 10:30 a.m. on Saturdays. There were no other classes on Saturday. I was the only female teacher conducting a class. Fearing for my safety, Daniel parked his car in a place where he could see the gym gate but no one else could see him. After Tai Chi class, he hid inside his car and waited until I locked the gate and got in my car to leave. What hurt him the most was that I only regarded him as an ordinary student and treated him as a younger brother. "I love her so much, but she never looks at me much. She didn't pay any attention to me at all. I'm very sad whenever she talks and laughs with other male students." He said to the two ladies whom he trusted. He also made them swear to keep his secret. The two ladies kept it a secret for him for several years. I really admire their honest promises and noble character towards Daniel.

In the summer of 2006, I finally learned about it. On one hand, I was very surprised; on the other hand, I felt really sorry for him. I had treated him as my student and a younger brother. I invited him and Gene to my daughter's house for Christmas. I even looked for girlfriends for him. At the same time, I began to observe him and test him. He was such a gentleman! He earned my admiration and trust.

Gene once had a bad cold and later it left him a bad allergy: every midnight, he began to have nasal congestion and he could not breathe. He had to sit up. After seeing the doctor and taking some tests, he was found to be allergic to the moss in the wall and the humidity in the air. He said he had to leave Monterey for health reasons. With the help of a friend we bought a manufactured home in Fremont in a beautiful senior park which is only for people who were over 55 years old. It was a quiet and beautiful place far from the coast and sunny all day long. Gene said he would move in first and let me retire and move in later.

We had to live apart in two cities. Occasionally he came down to visit me. Yet gradually, the feelings between us slowly faded. (Advice: husband and wife must not live separately).

Daniel was still the same as before, helping me drive my girlfriends to the Bay Area to watch shows, going to Chinese supermarkets to buy groceries, driving me to my Peking opera club activities and performances. When we returned from the Bay Area, he helped my friends bring large and small bags to their residences. He had no idea that I already knew the secret in his heart. Every time after driving me home, he politely said, "Have a good rest. I'm going home." One time my lumbar 5 which had been eaten by cancer cells and had a hole, was very sore after a day's exertion. I said, "Can you massage my back to reduce the pain?" He said, "Okay." He had practiced martial arts, taken classes on how to massage and had a training on how to care for patients in emergencies. After he gave me a massage, he asked me if I felt better and then, as usual, politely said,

"Have a good sleep. I'm going home." I was very touched for his well behaved manner. What a gentleman! I gradually respected him in my mind and my feelings towards him slowly changed.

What is love? It's hard to put into words. When a person is full oflove, there is like a small volcano in his heart, and the flame is always burning, which cannot be extinguished; uncontrollable. Love is a realm, an ideal, implemented in real life, but also a decision and choice. In the eyes of the world, I was thirteen years older than him, not so beautiful, and missing a breast. When Daniel first met me, he could see that I had purple spots on my face due to chemotherapy. My eyes were swollen. But in Daniel's eyes, I was his goddess. My spirit of fighting again cancer twice really impressed him. He was not afraid of talking to me about his frustration in his work, his conflicts with his girl friends and his worries of his sick mother etc.

My breakup with Gene was unexpected. Because we had been married for 16 years, we respected each other. Gene's father and stepmother lived in Portland, Oregon and his aunt lived in Eugene, Oregon. His brother's family lived near Seattle, Washington State and two of his best college classmates lived in Portland. We took my daughter Nancy traveling to stay in each home during the New Year's Holidays. In addition to visit the scenic spots in the two states, we also visited many other places, such as San Diego, Hawaii, Florida. Life was pleasant and calm. But there were no sparks in our life. Gene was an artist and painter who was loyal to his profession and had his own routine of everyday life. He ate no more than ten things and was not interested in anything else except to go to the beach to see boats and go home to paint the boat every day. He didn't go to bed until one or two o'clock in the morning. He could not tolerate noisy sounds or seeing dirty places. So when I went to my Peking opera clubs, he told me that the Peking Opera drumbeat was deafening his ears and gave him headaches. He apologized to me, saying that he could not go again. My activities, unless it was at my house, he was reluctant to participate. He treat me like a piece of art and for more than a decade without sexual desire.

After I broke up with him, I told a few of my Tai Chi students. They said, "We're not surprised at all. You two are already two horses running on two carriages." The scene at the time of the breakup was hard to believe. When I asked Gene that I wanted to break off my marriage agreement with him, he said, "Is it because I moved away?" He also asked me if we would still be friends in the future. In fact, I was also reluctant to let him go because of his unconditional love for me, his kindness and his gentleness. I knew the pain of leaving him would be unquestionable. I walked close to him and we hugged each other, both crying. After a few minutes, we both calmed down. I couldn't believe my ears.

He said, "I'd like you to go your own way. We don't need to go to the court. Tomorrow I'll go to the library and photocopy a document dissolving the marriage. After you and I sign it, I'll send it to the county office." No one could believe that Gene and I "divorced," and the issue was resolved so quietly. When I told Daniel about the dissolution of the marriage, he threw a tantrum with me angrily, "Who asked you to do this? From now on I will be a sinner and everyone will see me as a third wheel who has ruined your marriage..." I didn't expect Daniel react this way. I was also very angry with him and said, "It has nothing to do with you. Who said I was going to marry you? Now that I'm free, I can find any one I like. The two of us can break up, and you won't be guilty of that." But our feelings have been deeply rooted. Break up? It's easier said than done!

To make a long story short, after Gene and I dissolved our marriage, I respected him even more. When I went to my daughter's house to pass by Fremont, I often visited him and invited him to dinner. We still have close ties to this day. He also spoke regularly to Nancy and her two children, sending them his artwork. Gene had a heart surgery in 2015 and Daniel was going to accompany me to visit him. In the end I decided to fly alone to Oregon to take care of him for two weeks myself. Although we were no longer husband and wife, our friendship is eternal. This may also be incomprehensible to ordinary people. But it did happen between us. Up to now we two still communicate with emails.

In June 2008, Daniel and I went to the Bay Area to visit our daughter's family. When we passed by the Gilroy Outlets shopping center, Daniel said he was going to buy a pair of shoes. I suggested buying them on the way back but he insisted on buying them now. I said okay. When he got out of the car, he dragged me into the Zell Jewelry shop, pointed to the diamond counter and said, you pick one. I was really confused, thinking that my birthday was coming but I wouldn't need such an expensive gift. I pulled him to the door and asked him what he meant. He was embarrassed and said, "I want you to pick an engagement diamond ring."

I was not mentally prepared at all. I did not know how to answer. Later, the salesgirls gathered around and said, "We often saw women pulling men into the store to buy diamond rings, but we have seldom seen men pulling a woman into the store to buy diamond rings." This has become one of the stories that Daniel often told others. On Christmas 2008, Daniel and I flew to a beautiful island in Jamaica under the arrangement of our good friend Rena. A wonderful wedding was held in Jamaica. In 2009 Daniel's father, Arthur Dieli, took us to Sicily where Daniel's grandpa was born. It was considered our honeymoon. An unforgettable trip!

Although Gene and I were separated. He still cares about us as a loving father and old friends. When I first told him I was dating Daniel, I never expected him to say, "Then I'll be relieved. Daniel is a nice guy. He's taken care of you for years, I don't have to worry about you being alone in Monterey...." I was stunned that there was such a generous and kind man in the world! His love for me and his heart of gold gave me freedom. My friends hardly believe Gene is such a "generous gentleman." Some said, "Because he loves you unconditionally. As long as you are happy, he is happy. What a lucky woman I am!

Gene often sent Daniel and I cards of his new works. The birthday cards and holiday greeting cards that have flown in over the years have been made by his own hands. His greetings, whether given to me and Daniel or my daughter and her husband, grandson, granddaughter, are all created with his artistic genius. His love, his deep thoughts and feelings, and his care that he has cultivated over the years were in that artwork. What he sent was not cards, but his artistic genius, his kind heart and beautiful soul, the beauty he saw in the world, deep caring and selfless love. I also always send gifts on his birthday or holidays. When I had something good or successful, I also told Gene right away by email or phone. As before, he was happy for me from the bottom of his heart. For example, Daniel was going to work in Italy for three or four years. I decided to retire and go with him. Gene said, "What a great opportunity to see European culture, its long history, and the beautiful architecture and art with your own eyes."

Gene has a master's degree in painting and the history of European art. When the two of us were together, he took me to various museums, exhibitions, and explained the works of famous painters and the differences between them. I didn't understand, and dislike, the works of Picasso and Van Gogh at first. He explained them to me from the historical background and their outstanding artistic genius.

Why I am telling you about this is that a few weeks ago, paintings by these famous painters suddenly appeared in Carmel's shops. They were scarves from Germany, and tops from the United States. Some are printed on clothes, some are made of Cashmere material. I recognized them right away: Leonardo da Vinci in Italy, Picasso in Spain, Van Gogh in the Netherlands, Monet in France, and Renoir. Not considering the price, I bought four tops and four scarves at once. Without Gene's teachings, how could I have such an appreciation of that artwork? Every time I wear them, I think of the knowledge and artistic appreciation that heart of gold of Gene has given me. I have always enjoyed listening to the famous contemporary singers, love Western classical music, and know a little about it.

It was also nurtured by Gene's patient introduction and guidance. He was the mentor who led me into the Western culture. He is the giver of my spiritual food. After I bought an ideal property this year, I called him on the day it was closed. Then I thanked him for the way he opened all this up for me, and for the opportunities he created for me. Sincerely he congratulated Daniel and I on our success.

Let me introduce Daniel's family. His father was a full blooded Italian, born in Connecticut, USA, named Arthur Deli. He studied law, computers, and was proficient in several languages. He retired as a computer professor from a university in California. I had known him for 11 years and respected and admired him from the bottom of my heart. He was knowledgeable and well-learned. When he took us on a tour to Sicily for half a month, we met the relatives and residence of the Dieli family. Arthur tole me about the local history, culture, architecture, art, religion, etc. He passed away in California's capital, Sacramento, on March 19, 2019, at the age of 92. As he lay spending his last few hours, he endured with astonishing perseverance until Daniel and I rushed back from Italy, and then he passed away peacefully. As I mentioned in the beginning chapter, I've always been afraid of the dead. Even when my own father and mother died, I didn't dare to touch their bodies. But for some reason, I didn't have any feelings of fear for my father in-law's critically ill body. I was able to hold his hand and kiss his forehead. The wife of one of Daniel's cousins said to me, "You know what? Arthur told me when he was alive that he liked and valued you very much. He said you changed his son's fate." In 2013, Arthur led his fifth daughter Sara's entire family to San Mateo to see me perform Peking opera, "Farewell My Concubine" despite the fact that he had severe pain in his leg. I was so moved.

Daniel's grandfather was born in beautiful Sicily. He was a professional tuba player in the Lascar Opera Symphony Orchestra in Milan, Italy. Daniel majored in trumpet in college, but in the American Military Band he always played tuba. So the grandfather and Daniel had an unexplained connection.

After immigrating to Connecticut in the eastern United States, Daniel's grandfather opened a piano shop. The skill of craftsmanship was passed on to his sons and grandchildren (Daniel's father was so skillful that in his 80s, the tile floors of the entire room he lived in were installed by himself). Daniel was also a "handyman." He could fix anything: the carpentry work that our house needed, the electric problems needed to be fixed, even when my jewelry was broken, Daniel was able to fix it). His family's ancestors were not Sicilians, but a prominent family in northern Italy. No wonder he became more and more gentlemanly as he got older.

Daniel's mother was pure Irish. Her family immigrated to the eastern United States very early. His grandfather on the mother's side was a pardon lawyer appointed by five presidents of the United

States! Daniel's uncle also worked for the U.S. government and was a diplomat. He served in England and France. So his two daughters, one married to the Englishman and one to the Frenchman. Daniel and I visited both cousins when we were living in Vicenza , Italy.

When we visited them, we received a warm welcome. Daniel's mother was the youngest daughter. Her name was Alice, and she was very pretty. Her photo at 19 years of age looked just like a Hollywood movie star. Alice and Daniel's father, Arthur, met at the University of Georgia. Alice majored in English and Arthur studied law. Daniel told me that his dad's homework was often typed by Alice. The two fell in love with each other, and after getting married, they had a total of 7 children.

The night I first visited Daniel's dad, Arthur talked to me for a long time. He took out the photo albums he had collected for a lifetime, explaining them to me page by page. Among them were poems written in English by Alice. When he read them to me, he was so emotional that he had tears in his eyes. I said, "She was so beautiful and talented; you must have loved her very much."

Arthur said that although she passed away, "I felt like she was there for me every day." I was touched by his true feelings for his deceased wife. At the same time, I was also very pleased because he was a strong Italian man. It was not easy to show these nostalgic feelings for his wife in front of his children. I felt very lucky to be able to share his inner feelings as his new daughter in-law.

Daniel was the only boy. He has three older sisters and three younger sisters. After we got married, we had closer relationships with all of them.

I later learned that Daniel's parents adopted a Vietnamese orphan in addition to raising their own seven children. One can see that his parents were full of kindness and love for people. Daniel told me he never heard his parents argue. His father worked very hard from morning till night. His mother took care of the whole family: washing, cooking, cleaning up the house. The way she disciplined the children was very strict. Once she asked her eldest daughter and second daughter to put away their clothes. When after a few hours nothing was done, she opened the window and threw their clothes out. From then on everyone would fold their clothes neatly after the laundry was done.

When Daniel and I married, he always folded my clothes for me. No wonder! He also muttered, "I don't know if your mother taught you to fold clothes."

Sometimes I sleep later than him, and I found that he got up in the middle of the night to fold the clothes I took off. What interests me even more was that the clothes I wanted to wash, as long as they were not placed in the laundry basket, were always folded and neatly put away by him. He is such a meticulous gentleman. When we went to a restaurant, I put the used linen napkins on the table, and he would even fold those! At one point I couldn't help it, laughing and taking pictures of my used napkins, all neatly folded. I said that when I publish my autobiography in the future, I would put this photo in it.

Although I was not blessed to meet my mother-in-law, the image of her beauty and generosity, good family education, wisdom, her assistance to her husband, and her way of educating her children, remained vividly and deeply in my mind. The reason why Daniel has so many good qualities and disciplines was inextricably linked to his genes, family, and past lives. It seems that the two of us have a world of different personalities, but we have come together. Isn't that an incredible fate?

I just heard a story (April 6, 2022) that I would like to add here.

Daniel's second younger sister Sara and her husband Jorge came to visit us in Monterey for a short vacation. The four of us had a good time. After dinner when I asked Sara to look at the draft of my autobiography and the photos. When I talked about my regret that I hadn't the luck to meet her mom, she said, "Mom knows you." I was surprised and asked her, "How could it be? When Daniel and I were dating she already passed away." Sara said, "Daniel often talked to Mom about you. Once when I asked my mom how Daniel was doing lately, mom said he seems to like his Tai Chi teacher very much. He always told me how his Tai Chi teacher was. I wish the two of them could come together one day." Sara and I have known each other for over a decade. We get together a lot. She has two beautiful daughters. Both play the violin and spend the holidays with my grandchildren quite often. This was the first time we four adults got together without children. It was also the first time I had heard Sara talk about how his mother knew me. It can be seen that Daniel's hidden secret love was discovered by his mother. Isn't it a coincidence and providence that her hope had come true?

Anecdote:

The miracle of my bicycle front flip plus side flip accident demonstrated how Daniel took care of me and how I was protected by God.

In 2012, Daniel and I, with the help of a real estate specialist, Ms. Bamboo, bought a condo that was below market value in an excellent location-Pebble Beach. Pebble Beach is a world-famous golf course park with four world-class golf courses, three five star hotels, and 4,530 homes with a population of 9,036, with an average age of 65 years old (which is almost the same situation where I live now-Rossmoor in Walnut Creek California). It is also known as Del Monte forest. The vast majority are of white race. It was a beautiful location, full of pine trees, with the famous 17-Mile Drive and other tourist attractions.

Monterey has a long history. Many Guangdong immigrants settled here around 1850, forming a Chinese fishing colony. They caught abalone and squid. In old times, the girls sold sparkling pebbles they found from the seashore as ornamental gifts. The success of the coastal Chinese in Monterey was envied and hated by the non-Chinese race who once set fire to the Chinese residential areas. As a result, many Chinese had to move to San Francisco. Before I published this bool, I saw the City Council of Monterey formally took responsibility for the fire in 1906 and apologized to the victims of the fire and their descendants, as well as to the Chinese who had been discriminated against for half a century. At the time San Francisco had just 108 people, Monterey was already the capital of California.

When I first arrived at Monterey, I fell in love with this small coastal city. I didn't know why, but I just thought that the taste of this small coastal town had a special flavor. The architecture, the streets, the scenery, the climate, and even the air had an attraction to me. It is a blessing to live in this small coastal haven, just 120 kilometers south of San Francisco and 320 kilometers away from Los Angeles. It is a blessing to be able to live in an upscale residential area. Not only is the 17-mile tour drive, an attractive tourist place, but many cyclists also come here for to cycle on weekends. We often see colorful groups of cyclists drive by our front windows.

October 13, 2013, it was a Saturday which was also the Chinese Chong Yang Festival (According to traditional Chinese custom, it is the day when people climb to higher places to overlook the scenery to be considered Senior Day).

On a whim, I proposed Daniel and I ride our bikes around the Pebble Beach. Putting on our newly purchased sportswear, drawing up the route, we both set off. When I was working in Beijing, I rode and traveled by bicycle almost every day. The feeling of being free to ride here was very pleasant. I once drove by bicycle from my home in Xiaoshiqiao (the central Axis of Beijing) to the Ming Tombs for a day with my college classmates, a round trip of about 111 miles. Very few girls could make that trip. I was athletic and a good biker.

Reaching a stop sign, Daniel stopped and waited for me. Because it was a turn and a rather steep downhill ahead, I squeezed the brake with my right hand, forgetting that it was the front brake. When I swung my right leg off the bike, I suddenly lost control of my body. Before I realized it, my body was thrown right off the bike, and I lost consciousness. Fortunately, that day at Daniel's request, I wore my helmet. From the damage to the front handle of the bike and the recesses on my helmet, it was estimated that I had a front flip, and then a side flip. Anyway, I lost consciousness when I was in the air. Daniel only heard a snap, and by the time he looked back, I was lying on my back on the left side of the bike unconscious!

What happened next was what Daniel told me: he hurried to my side and saw me lying on the road, he was lost, and called my name again and again. Just then two cars drove by, a man and a woman, both stopped. It turned out that they were nurses at CHOMP (the nearby hospital) who had just finished their shift. (Daniel later joked with his friends that Lydia was so blessed that if I had fallen, no one would have come over until I woke up myself.) The nurses immediately called an ambulance and the first responder gave me first aid. I woke up and asked Daniel what had happened. The paramedic said, "Ma'am, you just fell off the bike." I said, "I didn't ride a bike," obviously disoriented and confused by my experience.

Sentence after sentence I repeatedly asked, "Daniel, where are we? Where are we?" At that time, my high blood pressure reached

200, and they judged that I might have a brain damage. I was conscious but not coherent. Although there was a big hospital nearby (CHOMP), there was no head trauma center. They decided to send me to the head trauma center in Santa Clara with a helicopter. By this time I was basically awake. Hearing the helicopter right next to me. There were only two ambulance crew seats and a place for me. They told Daniel to drive himself to the trauma center in Santa Clara.

Probably more than 20 minutes later, someone carried me off the helicopter and took me into the emergency room. I didn't know what they did, but when I was sent to the ward, I immediately threw up. My left arm hurt badly, and the inside of upper left arm hurt terribly. The final diagnosis was that my lips and the back of my hand had been scratched, but there was no fracture. There was a slight concussion. They gave me a painkiller.

Then I heard the nurse say that my daughter was on the phone. It turned out that Daniel immediately called Nancy. I answered the call from my daughter and told her I was okay. She had planned to drive over from the Bay Area, but thankfully she made the phone call first, because her husband was on a business trip. Her 2-year-old daughter and 7-year-old son were both at home. It might be very difficult for her. When she heard that I was okay, she needn't to drive over.

I put the phone down when I heard Daniel's voice, "Where is Lydia? Where is Lydia?" I saw his anxious face looking for me from room to room. I shouted, "I am here!" He made three steps into two steps and rushed to my bedside. When he saw that I was fine, with a big sigh, he said, "Oh my God! You are okay." Then he told me in detail how he saw me lying on the ground, unconscious, and all the details of what happened afterwards. Before he came to the hospital, he also called his father, second younger sister, Sara, and Nancy. I said, "You don't have to alarm so many people and make them all worry about me." He said, "You don't know how bad you were and how scared I was. In case something happened to you, I would not know what to do "

Later, the doctor observed me for more than an hour. The traffic police also came in and asked me many questions. With a very serious expression on his face and a very stiff tone as if I had committed some crime. I thought to myself, he didn't have any sympathy. I just had such a big accident, but he didn't seem to care at all. The way he asked me was like interrogating a prisoner. Fortunately, my mind was still relatively clear. I answered all his questions. I also signed a form. He didn't say a word and left.

I asked the doctor if we could go home. I was happy to hear the doctor say, "Yes. you may go home now. If you have questions, you can call us right away." Relieved, Daniel happily drove me home.

The next day Daniel went to the office of the director of my department and told him what happened. The director didn't tell anyone either. That gave me a good rest for a week. Daniel checked on me every now and then from his office and took care ofme.

Later, my friends slowly all heard about my accident. My eldest cousin said, "You're so lucky. That kind of fall might have been a terrible accident. It could bring crushing fractures for anyone. You didn't even have a single bone broken."

What a miracle! I thank God, I thank my gate keeper! I thank my guardian angel! In addition, I would like to thank the dance teachers, martial arts teachers, and sports teachers, who have nurtured me over the years. It is precisely because I am usually very active, flexible and responsive, so I did not have a big disaster at that critical moment. In short, I think if one has great love in his/her heart and always feels grateful, he/she will receive the protection of the universe and the help of God at a certain time of crisis. I certainly did.

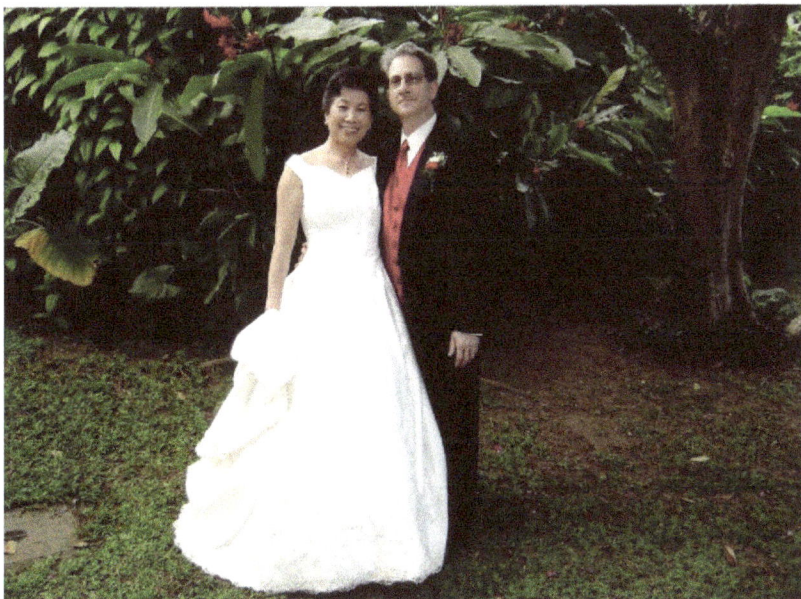

Daniel and I got married in a resort in Jamaica

Chapter 18

Daniel's Struggle with the Disease

July 7, 2022 at the Pacific Cancer Center in Monterey, California, Dr. Zhang, a Chinese-American oncologist, made an exception for the four of us (Daniel's eldest sister, second younger sister, and I) to enter a conference room in the center (usually only one person is allowed to accompany the patient). She turned on the computer and put on the screen the CT scan Daniel took on June 16. When I first met Dr. Zhang on June 30, she had already shown Daniel and I the CT scan results. Now she said very seriously, "I sent Daniel to be hospitalized on June 30, and had the biopsy on July 1. Now the results have come out."

She pointed to the stereoscopic image on the screen and said, "You see, two tumors on his pancreas have metastasized to many places in his liver. My diagnosis turned out to be a stage IV patient with pancreatic cancer. The cancer has metastasized to most parts of the liver. Without chemotherapy, he can live for 1 to 3 months. If going though chemotherapy he can live for about a year. Of course this is only the mean number which may change a little."

Suddenly, the air in the conference room seemed to freeze and there was a dead silence. Although on the night of June 30, when I told my eldest cousin, who had been the director of the oncology department of the Beijing Air Force General Hospital about Daniel's hospitalization for a biopsy, she decisively told me: "I don't have to wait for his biopsy results. I have concluded that Daniel has metastatic pancreatic cancer." But now when I heard Dr. Zhang's clear answer, I was still shocked and dumbfounded.

We all saw that Daniel didn't say a word. He took out the handkerchief from his pocket and wiped the beads of sweat from his forehead. Daniel's eldest and the second younger sister asked Dr. Zhang a few questions and within a few minutes the four of us silently left the "Pacific Cancer Center" and drove to Del Monte shopping center to get some medicine for Daniel. Since they drove to the cancer center directly from Bay area, I led the way. I had no idea why I couldn't find Del Monte shopping center! I drove around and around and finally I found it. On the surface I was very calm, but I knew I was lost and confused by what we had learned.

In the center, our eldest sister Lisa said, "Daniel's illness is in an advanced stage. I don't know whether it is worth going through chemotherapy and that horrible suffering. Let's have a meeting to discuss it."

For some reason, we didn't have that meeting. The two sisters were busy leaving. At this time, Dr. Zhang had arranged for Daniel to start chemotherapy next Tuesday. After a while, she called again and said, "I don't want to delay any longer, so I have arranged to start chemotherapy next Monday, once every two weeks, for a total of 8 times." I thanked Dr. Zhang for her promptness and decisiveness as if Daniel's family doctor's delay before had been remedied. I hoped that Daniel's life would be saved, but I couldn't help my bitter tears.

I knew Daniel had been feeling sick since May 2022. When he went to see his family doctor, the old lady doctor kept delaying any process to Daniel's condition. At the beginning of June, she asked him to do an ultrasound, thinking that there was a problem with the gallbladder. Nothing was found wrong there. Then she asked him to have an MRI on June 10. It was found that there were two small tumors in the liver and there was a tumor on the pancreas, but she did not pay attention to it. It was dragged out to June 16 for a CT scan. The radiologist had suspected that it was pancreatic cancer, but it was dragged out until June 30 to find Dr. Zhang of the Pacific Cancer Center! More than a month had passed!

No treatment was given to the patient in that interval. These are the problems with the U. S. medical system. Doctors are very critical to patients. It is a matter of life and death. This doctor did not fulfill her duty. I only learned these results later when I asked for pathological examination results from the oncologist Dr.Zhang. Before meeting Dr. Zhang, every time I asked Daniel if he could let me go with him to see his family doctor, he wouldn't let me go to see the old lady, his family doctor. When I asked him for the results of the MRI and CT scans, he said that the results were in the family doctor's office, and he didn't have them. (According to American medical rules, only the patient can ask for a copy of his medical records. So I could not see the results). The MRI and CT scan results were printed out later when Daniel and I first met Dr. Zhang in person.

During Daniel's back and forth examination, a strange event happened: Unexpectedly, his family doctor died suddenly on June 27! After hearing all this, my eldest cousin said angrily, "She deserves it! At the time, it was found that there was a problem with Daniel's pancreas, immediate measures should be taken right away. How can they let the patient wait for more than a month! When I was a doctor, when I saw this kind of report I would take action on the same day. How come American doctors allow a patient with a pancreatic problem wait more than a month! They are making a mockery of human's life!" Whatever, it was too late.

Of course, cancer doesn't form in one day. Daniel had been working for more than a dozen hours a day for years (consciously working overtime without being paid). Even on weekends, he often went to the office to work overtime without telling anybody. This time he had cancer, had to take sick leave, and went through retirement procedures, but he still asked me to drive him to his office and spend more than three hours explaining his work procedures and teaching his subordinate staff. When he left, everyone came out to see him off. He said to me, "It is not easier to work so hard today, but later it will be a lot easier for them to catch up. I hope they won't' have the problem I ran into last summer: My boss was angry with the supervisors, even though we were also friends, she did not explain anything to me and just walked out. I was in the dark about that for many months." I still vividly remembered that during that time, Daniel was really stressed out and quite restless. Seeing that he was now considerate of others despite of his own serious illness and suffering, a high respect for him arose in my heart, but I felt very sad at the same time.

Daniel indeed deserved the nickname I gave him: "The loyal soldier of our party." Many of my Chinese friends know his nickname. Writing all this, I want to tell everyone that life and health are more important than anything else! I have witnessed the harsh reality that my husband was suffering day and night in a world where science and technology are so advanced, as the United States is the world's leading scientific and technological country. The sacred duty of a doctor is to cure the sick and save the lives of people. Now I see the patient's trust in the doctor is sometimes tarnished. His family doctor had been negligent. I wonder how many other people had the same miserable experience. So I appeal to our society to change this situation!

Three chemotherapy treatments from July 11 to August 8 tortured Daniel immensely. On August 11th he told me that he had decided not to have any further treatments. I was also a metastatic patient with stage IV breast cancer 22 years ago. An invasive malignant breast cancer discovered in 2000 and metastasized to 7 parts of my bones in 2002, including one on the right skull. I had two rounds of chemotherapy, four times in each round, and the side effects and bad consequences are still fresh in my memory. Even today, I feel terrible and chilled when I think about it. I understood Danial's pain and his decision all too well. Pancreatic cancer is the king of all cancers. The hope for a cure is very slim. However, if you don't do chemotherapy, you will give up treatment. There is no hope at all. It is a great pity that chemotherapy is also very devastating to the human body. Maybe from the beginning, Daniel shouldn't have started the chemo and would have suffered less. I thought about it back and forth, but I couldn't figure it out whether he should stop the chemo treatment

That Day when Daniel told me he won't have any further chemo, I couldn't sleep until after 12 o'clock in the middle of the night. The more I thought about it, the sadder I became. I was helpless, but i did not want to see him endure the pain day and night. Soon he might leave me. I hadn't cried since he fell ill because I was busy shopping every day, making him nutritious soups, taking him back and forth between the hospital, chemotherapy center, and pharmacy; receiving many visits from his 5 sisters, worrying about how to discuss this with my two granddaughters, who were very close with him. I could not bear to tell them that Daniel was dying of pancreatic cancer. My suppressed emotions, that had been held in check for several weeks, suddenly erupted like a volcano. I began to cry loudly and tears were like a river running down my cheeks.

I never imagined that Daniel would be so calm in the face of such news about his health. He took my hand and said, "Don't be so hysterical. Have you forgotten what you told me how your friend in

Guizhou mountain said, 'Don't be overjoyed when you're happy. Don't cry when you're sad. It's midnight now, go to bed!" I took his hand and sobbed for a while, confused, and finally fell asleep.

On August 12, the eldest sister Lisa visited us for the fifth time from Sacramento, the capital of California. She worked in the U.S. Army for many years and retired as a Major. She later studied for a Ph.D. and became a professor in a university computer lab. She had five younger sisters, and one younger brother, Daniel. Her Mom and Dad trained her to be in charge of her 6 siblings. As a result, she was extremely capable. She spent another three hours helping transfer all Daniel's accounts, credit cards, etc. to my name, and reset all the usernames and passwords. Daniel and I were very grateful.

Every time Lisa came for a few hours, she helped us to sort out computer files. Under the pretext of sensitive stomach, she didn't eat or drink. I told her I knew where Daniel's dedication came from. Because no matter what Daniel was asked to do, he wouldn't eat or drink until everything was done. I called him "Camel." After the eldest sister left in the afternoon, my daughter's family came to visit us in the evening with chicken and duck meat dishes and Ganoderma lucidum, an herb associated with longevity in China. As mentioned earlier, Daniel and my daughter's family were very close, especially the two children who were unrestrained with him, and he loved them dearly. I knew that the two would lose Daniel before they grew up. Watching them affectionately together, my tears came down my cheeks, but I was afraid of darkening everyone's mood, so I had to quietly walk away and secretly wipe away the tears.

The next day, it was Saturday, August 13. After dinner, Daniel asked everyone sit around the dinner table with a legal sized yellow pad in his hand and began reading the "farewell letter" he had written to everyone on October 16, 2021 (his birthday was October 17) last year. He couldn't help sobbing as he was reading. We all couldn't' help shedding tears. He wrote a total of 10 pages in pencil. What he wrote to everyone were words from his heart. His feelings were so sincere, the meaning was so far-reaching. All in all the words were so touching. In the letter he wrote his inside observations and thanks for everyone, his sincere feelings and hopes, and even apologies.

From Daniel, I learned what is the true meaning of life, and what is loving and sincere. The difference in our humanity is in the soul. His characteristic calm, and strong perseverance in the fight against the disease moved me to tears from time to time.

I remembered when his stomach hurt badly, he joked, "I now know what it's like for a woman to have a baby." One night, his pain began to hit him again (the painkillers worked for only 12 hours). He said, "Lydia, it is coming! Is it a boy or a girl?" I laughed bitterly and shouted, "It is a twin!" Facing the illness, he was still so humorous and witty, which showed his inner strength and optimistic attitude.

Since Daniel was officially diagnosed with stage IV metastatic pancreatic cancer to his liver on July 7, his five sisters and my daughter's family have taken turns to see him many times. Each time he spent 2 to 4 hours without pause to tell his military training stories to them with photo albums, from joining the army to serving in South Korea three times with his military band; to service in Germany; to aid for Haiti; to parachute training (after three arduous trainings to finally become Jump Master and Jump Master Trainer; then participating in special forces missions. He had such an incredible memory. He told stories reminiscing about his upbringing in the upstate New York and Washington D.C. areas; the story of his learning to practice with different martial arts masters. Sometimes he stands in front of the shrine I bought for him and explains the essence and purpose of

Tantric Buddhism and Pure Land Buddhism. He introduced the name and background story of each Buddha statue he brought home and the story of each Thangka. He told the stories from the various books he had read to discuss with any "guest," or even watched a scene of his favorite TV series with the "guest," and then aired his opinion.

The tea I made for the guests or the meals I cooked were cold and he had no time to let the guests eat or drink. I watched him turn into a "talker" in front of our guests. I worried he would be too tired because our guests were too polite to stop him. But I was also impressed by his "encyclopedic" talent. Although I have listened to his stories several times, I felt happy for him. He has the energy and interest to explain his "success" experiences. He swept away the wrong conclusions about himself that "he was a failure," that he "let his father down," and "was the most unsuccessful in the family." Never have I seen him so proud of himself.

I will now translate the contents of the "farewell letter" he wrote to each of my daughter's family here.

His headline was:

"Dan's Perspective of the Chen Family"

"Thank you for allowing me to be part of your family."

Here is what Daniel wrote for me:

"Dear Lydia Olson (Li Xianghui): Here I quote a passage from the American TV series The Kaminsky Method: 'We have been husbands and wives for 13 years. During this time, I never failed to love you. I've been angry with you, confused by you, and even hurt by you, but I've always loved you. You are the woman I was looking for from the beginning'.

This is a passage that Alan, a character in the TV show said at his wife's funeral. Although this is what another character said, it represents my feelings for you as well. No one can replace you. You are the lady I've been looking for since the beginning. I know I'm not always so amiable, kind and noble, sometimes downright unfriendly and obnoxious, but I didn't mean it, and that doesn't represent my true feelings for you at all. The real emotions are - sincere love, affectionate love, a sense of happiness, and a sense of safety and security - and these were things I lacked all my life before I met you."

Signed by Daniel on

August 13, 2022

I was listening to him. I hugged him and cried. My granddaughter Audrey came to hold us both. My son-in-law hinted that his son had videotaped Daniel's reading the letter from the beginning (I typed his handwritten English into text that night and saved it on the computer). Daniel, exhausted after reading the five letters to each one of us, said, "I find it very embarrassing to read this to you. But that's what I've always wanted to say. I'm so tired, I'm going to bed."

After my granddaughter and I sent him back to the bedroom, we both went into the jacuzzi in the backyard. Every time my daughter brought her in, it was the most enjoyable time for both of us. What I can't understand is that these were all written by Daniel on October 16 last year, the day before his 63rd birthday, how could he have a premonition last year that he would not live long? Looking at the black sky, I said sadly: "Tong tong (my granddaughter's Chinese name), Daniel will not live long, I am so sad." I was really surprised by the words that this ten-year-old girl comforted me. She said them so naturally and fluently and even with a little smile on her face. I couldn't believe my ears! She said, "Grandma, don't be sad. Daniel is never going to leave us. Even when he leaves us, his spirit and soul are with us forever. When we meet him again, he will have a new and healthier body. Maybe we won't recognize him anymore. If Daniel leaves us, he will be going to heaven. He will no longer be in pain and will live a more enjoyable life. He doesn't have to pay any taxes anymore. He will also protect us in heaven and will take good care of us. His spirit and soul will never leave you. He will bless us from any danger!"

Looking at her innocently beautiful and smiling little face, I was stunned! I asked her where she had heard or learned it, and if she had been to church. She smiled and said, "I haven't been to any church." I asked her again if her friend had told her about it. She said no, no one told me about it. That's what I thought. I held her tightly in my arms, letting the waves in the hot tub wash against us both, letting the red, blue, and orange lights in the water change color in flashes, looking at the deep blue sky of night and the swaying pine branches around us, my heart gradually quieted down. Before Tong tong went to bed (she always sleeps with me whenever we meet) she ran to Daniel's bedside and told him what she had said to me in the hot tub.

The next morning I pleasantly told my son-in-law and my daughter how Tong tong comforted me with surprising words. My son-in-law said to his daughter, "Now you should write down everything you said to grandmother yesterday." I gave Tong tong a piece of paper and a pencil. She stood at the table near the entrance to the door and wrote half page English text beautifully. The content is the same as what I recorded above. Then she walked over to Daniel and showed him what she had just written. I hurriedly took a picture of her beautifully handwritten page and saved it on my phone. I was always worried that the children would not be able to handle news of

Daniel's fatal disease, but what I did not expect was that she enlightened me and comforted me. My heart is much calmer. No matter how long Daniel's life span is, I will definitely do my best to accompany him, carefully make him a nutritious soup every day, and repay his care and selfless love for me over the years!

Daniel knew his life wouldn't last long. He wanted to do as much as possible for me in the last days of his life. These days he also used amazing perseverance to help me clean the windows of my car and repair my earring and a flower that fell from my slippers. From time to time, he also went out to clean the pine needles by the pool and even wiped the inside and outside of the cooking stove. Sometimes he also helped me wash pots and dishes. I admired him from my heart, admired his courage to fight with pain every day, chanting sutras with Buddhist beads, reading books, watching TV, and sometimes Zhan Zhuang (standing meditation). He is ready to leave this earthly world without fear. I watched him silently, sometimes secretly taking pictures or videos. The tears in my heart would be the source of my memory of his good qualities.

On Tuesday, August 16th, Daniel's second younger sister, Sara, and her family of four came to visit us for the second time in Monterey (Sara herself had been here four times). Under the influence of Daniel's grandfather and parents, the six daughters and a son each learned one or two musical instruments. The eldest sister often organizes family concerts. Daniel will give his trumpet to Sara. But he was afraid that she would not be able to play well, so he gave her a demonstration. I was preparing snacks for them in the kitchen when I heard the beautiful sound of trumpets. I opened Daniel's Buddhist and computer room. I was surprised to see that it was Daniel playing the trumpet! I immediately found my phone and recorded the touching scene.

Three years ago, Daniel used the trumpet to say good-bye to his deceased father. Unexpectedly, this scene reappeared. Daniel picked up the trumpet, and I felt as if he was saying good-bye with its music to us. The piece he blew was Russian composer Dmitry Shostakovich's Paris Jazz Suite No. 2 Waltz Round Dance, a brisk dance piece. How could a patient with stage IV pancreatic cancer, whose cancer cells had metastasized to most of the liver and had gone through three rounds of chemotherapy have the strength and perseverance to play the trumpet?! The sound of Daniel's trumpet was intermittent. Daniel's words to me several times now are ringing in my ears: "My head seems always stuffed with cotton and my ears are always buzzing. I felt extremely bad. When I left this world, all of you were all crying around me, but my soul already left my body. I am in the sky overlooking you grieving for me. I will take care of you in heaven and bless you."

Daniel's trumpet was holy and solemn, full of strength and hope, leading me to forget my pain, and stand on the high ground of the soul, merging into the eternal realm of life. Daniel's trumpet echoed in the room for a long time, reverberated in our hearts, and lingered for a long time in the sky over our house.

Today is September 27, 2022. I am finishing my autobiography in English version, Daniel still is still hanging there: meditation every day, reading heart sutra and other Buddhist sutra, watching TV, receiving visitors, and cleaning the yard once a while. I don't know how long his life span will last but I am still with him.

The whole October was a roller coaster for both Daniel and me. It seemed he was getting better and we chose to make a miracle happen. However, it didn't go the way we hoped. His pain level was getting worse and had to use morphine from time to time. His dharma sister Susan Scheck tried to come every day to do sitting meditation with him and invited me to join them. She was one of my Tai Chi students too when I was teaching at local community college 20 years ago. She is 91 years old now and loves Daniel like his mother. Daniel and Susan studied Tibetan Buddhism together for quite a few years. We were both surprised by her boundless energy and sincere desire to help people. I was really grateful for her coming to our house almost every day. It was real quality time for Daniel to concentrate on his practice of meditation. I also believed Daniel drew strength from the limited time he had in this world.

On October 17, 2022 Daniel survived his 64 birthday. On Oct. 22 my good friends Xiao yan and her husband David Zhang held a birthday celebration for Daniel and David in their home (Those two men were born on the same years and same month only two days apart). Another couple of our friends, Tom Wang and his wife An Li also joined us. Tom also prepared a beautiful photo and video show of our three family trips over the past few years, such as to Lake Tahoe, Alaska and Eastern Europe. None of us believed that we looked so young then. At first Daniel didn't think he was able to attend the birthday party, but he tried to make it. He even reparked our car because he didn't like the location I parked.

Whoever thought that his brain lost function the next day, Sunday, Oct. 23, when my friend Jane came to visit him. He did talk to Jane as a normal person but he said there was another girl sitting at the dining table with us and urged me to talk to her. I was shocked to notice his brain deteriorated so fast. On Tuesday morning Oct. 25 at 4:30 am, Daniel woke me up and showed me a message on his cell phone. He didn't understand what it meant. I saw he typed a whole bunch of letters on his message and tried to send them out. "What does it mean?" he asked me. I told him it was he who typed it. At the same time he felt frustrated that he could not read who sent him messages.

I knew immediately that the cancer cells had attached to his brain badly. I reported his strange behavior to all his five sisters right away.

At 8 am, he got up and told me nobody was at work and he had to go to his office. I told him he had retired and had nothing to do with his office. It was very scaring to see him lose his mind in such a short time. Luckily his third elder sister bought an airline ticket right away and told me she would fly from the east coast to Monterey the next day. On Wednesday morning, Oct. 26, Daniel told me the deputy asked him to have a meeting. I was frustrated to see him still so involved with his work and not in his right mind. I was counting every minute to wait for Annamaria to arrive.

When Annamaria walked into our house at 2:10 in the afternoon, Daniel could not recognize his closest elder sister. That night he could not walk anymore.

We reported all this to the hospice. Deitra, the caring nurse who had been taking care of Daniel over the last two months, found him a bed to be hospitalized on Friday, October 29.

On Friday Daniel had already lost his consciousness, but he looked so relaxed in the hospice bed when I told him the nurses were taking care of him now. The nurse told me before a patient passed away the last organ to lose function was his hearing. So I told him from time to time that he didn't have to worry about me. His second younger sister Sara came to Monterey on Friday to be with us. When I took Annamaria to the airport on Saturday morning, she told me Daniel and the two elder sisters had already arranged everything after his passing away without bothering me: There will be no farewell to his remains or any funeral ceremony. Daniel told his sisters, "Lydia can buy houses and cars but she cannot handle my passing away. Please don't involve her after I am gone." I was very touched by his deep consideration. Annamaria told me that after the cremation at the local Paul Mortuary his ashes would be shipped to the Mortuary in Gloucester, Massachusetts, where his grandfather bought a cemetery for the Dieli's family. He will be buried with his grandparents, his parents, and his second elder sister Mary. He also told his two older sisters, "I don't want Lydia to be involved with my death. Please help me to manage all the paperwork as I left everything of mine to her."

What a loving and considering husband! I hold Annamaria and we both cried.

On Sunday noon, Oct. 30, Daniel's youngest sister, Nancy Dieli, flew in from Dallas and visited her loving older brother for the last time.

Sara said she didn't feel right that on Sunday afternoon, Daniel would be all by himself that night. I said I would stay with him in his room.

The nurses brought in a folding bed for me. I held Daniel's hand and told him to his ear that I would be with him that night. He seemed to understand me. The nurses came in every one or two hours to give him morphine. By 6 o'clock in the morning, I felt asleep. Somebody touched my shoulder at 6:35 a.m. I woke up and the nurse told me, "He is gone." I set up right away and asked him, "When?" He said, "Just a minute ago."

I didn't expect that Daniel would leave the world so fast. He stopped breathing. He had no pain. I remembered he told me, "When I am gone, don't cry. I don't want to come back to this world again. If you cry, I will be attached to you and I cannot go to heaven." I said jokingly, "Then I won't cry I will celebrate you're going to heaven." He said, "You can cry a little bit, otherwise other people will feel strange that your husband died and you didn't cry. You can be sad for two days, and then find a day to have your friends come together and

entertain them with a nice meal." I didn't expect this day would come so soon, only three nights after he was hospitalized.

I was thankful for my good friend Katie Wang the previous day. She reminded me to prepare a set of Tai Chi outfits for Daniel when he passed away. I told the nurses that I had to rush home to get his funeral outfit. Getting out of the hospice building, I thanked Sara and God for giving me a chance to spend the last night with my beloved Daniel. He was so kind that he left us without any bother. My heart jumped fast but I didn't cry right away. The nurse asked me whether I would be oaky to drive home to get the clothes by myself. I told him that I would be fine, and I would be careful driving home.

I got in my car, a little bit shaking, but I thought of the words Daniel told me and I was grateful that he won't suffer anymore. I prayed loudly from time to time, "Amituofo! Oh Ma Ni Pe Mei Hong! Gate Gate Paragate Parasamgate, Bodhi Svaha!"

In the darkness, I didn't cry. I tried to calm myself down.

I tried to help him go to heaven.

I came home and told Sara that Daniel just left us. I picked up the most beautiful Tai Chi outfit and a pair of Tai Chi boots he often wore. We came back to his side. The nurses and Sara helped to put on the Tai Chi outfit for him. One of the nurses told me she had never see such a beautiful and embroidered outfit before.

In less than two hours, Kevin from Paul Mortuary arrived. He asked, "Who is Lydia?" I said, It is me." He politely asked, "Can I give you a hug?" I said, "Yes." I don't remember now what he said. However, I remembered he stood at the foot of Danie's bed, raised his right hand in salute to Daniel. He said, "Sir, thank you for your services to our country!" My tears came down, but I swallowed the sorrow back. He also brought a National Flag to cover Daniel's body when he would take him away. I requested to cover Daniel's body with a flag when he was still in bed. I took a short video and a photo. I think Daniel would like it. I was so proud of him!

I never saw Daniel again.

Sara took care of everything afterwards. Sara and I went home. I suddenly understood what my friend Nancy Zhu told me. When she visited Daniel in October two weeks before Daniel passed away, I told her I would rent part of the house, otherwise I would feel so lonely. She said, "You might change your mind after he is really gone." She is absolutely right. When Sara helped me to clear the house, I changed my mind. The house seemed completely empty without Daniel. His love was everywhere, and I will carry it with me the rest of my life. However, I can never live in that house again.

Daniel was buried on Dec. 16, 2022, in Gloucester, Massachusetts, by the local Veterans Bureau. It was a rainy and windy day. His third eider's whole family and his second younger sister Paula were all there. The ceremony was recorded by his nephew. The Bureau sent several military officers. The bugle was playing outside the tent while they put an American National Flag over the vase of his ashes. And then two officers folded the national flag and presented to Paula. Daniel instructed his sisters that Lydia would not participate the ceremony. I thank him being so thoughtful, because he knew I would be so sad that something might happen to me.

I will definitely visit him after 2 or 3 years when I am ready.

Daniel is gone physically but his love for me, his blessing for me are forever there. Our souls are deeply connected. I hanged the beautifully framed photos of our marriage in my new bedroom. Looking at the lovely photos, I know he is still with me everyday.

Obituary from the newspaper in Monterey

DANIEL MICHAEL DIEL!
Oct. 17, 1958 v Oct. 31, 2022

Daniel Michael Dieli, former resident of Pebble Beach, passed away at the age of 64, in the company of his family. Dan's sense of adventure, and the stories he told with a marvelous wit will be treasured by his wife, Lydia Xianghui Li Olson; her daughter, Nancy Xiao nan Wang and son-in-law Chi Chen; his sisters, Alice L. Dieli, Annamaria D. Colburn and her husband Dustin Colburn, Paula C. Dieli and her husband Michael Schubert, Sara C. Dieli and her husband Jorge Gomez, and Nancy E. Dieli; as well as two grandchildren; six nieces and nephews and a grandniece and grand-nephew. He was preceded in death by his parents, Arthur and Alice Dieli; and his sister, Mary A. Dieli.

Dan was born in Washington, D.C. and lived in Maryland before moving with his parents and sisters to Henderson Harbor, New York, where he spent weekends working alongside his father to renovate the family's home or work on projects at the schools that he and his sisters attended.

Dan learned to play the trumpet in high school, and developed a lifelong love of the instrument. He graduated with a BA in music education from the Crane School of Music at SUNY, Potsdam in 1980, specializing in the tuba. After he graduated, uninspired by the prospects of following the path as a music teacher, he decided "for the first time in my life to do exactly what my father recommended and join the Army band," while he took tuba lessons from a member of the New York Philharmonic Orchestra at the same time. He graduated from Army basic training in 1980 and then served with the Army band in Brooklyn, Germany, San Francisco, and in Seoul, South Korea.

Never one to pass over any challenge, Dan attended the Army's Special Forces Assessment and Selection (SPAS) training, where he was nicknamed "Bandman" by his teammates. He was selected to continue his special forces training, and earned his airborne qualifications, and later completed Jump Master school. His stories from this time in his life, in which he always noted that "names and dates were changed to protect the innocent," were humorous and ironic, eschewing tales of grueling training in favor of the legend of an airborne school classmate who was "bad luck," a label that Dan scoffed at until he learned first-hand what it felt like to be knocked unconscious mid-jump. Dan's military awards and decorations included the Meritorious Service Medal, Army Commendation Medal (3rd award), Army Achievement Medal (2nd award), and Senior Parachutist Badge, among others.

Dan was protective of his parents and six sisters, and when he visited family, he often found himself pulled toward house repairs or refinishing furniture ifleft unsupervised. After taking an early retirement from the Army, Dan continued as a civilian employee for the Department of Defense, and continued a lifelong study of the martial arts, earning his second-degree black belt from the Korean Hapkido Federation. He will be greatly missed by all of us who loved him.

Dan and his family appreciate the care and support from the Pacific Cancer Care Center, the Hospice of the Central Coast, and the Paul Mortuary.

As my granddaughter Audrey told me,
I, too, feel Daniel is with me everyday.

Chapter 19

Friends Are the Companions of My Soul

November the 10th, upon the invitation of Grace Wang, I drove to Rossmoor, a beautiful over 55-ye2D. degrees from Wayne State University in Michigan. Because of their far-sighted view and hard work, they became billionaires.

Instead of spending the money for themselves, they donated and supported many organizations and students. So, the couple was well-respected in many areas. Unfortunately, Peter passed away at the age of 83 and I was honored to be invited to stay with Grace.

She has such a big heart, big love, and cares for everyone around her. In today's demoralized new world, people's minds have been polluted to an extent that we feel heartbroken. However, while I lost my dear husband and suffered an irreparable mental trauma, Grace surrounded me with her sincere friendship, deep love and true caring.

Jane Shaw, my long time good friend and co-worker, table tennis partner, and travel companion, booked back-to-back cruise tours. Those two ladies helped me to get out of the misery and suffering of being lost. Their companionship and warmth changed me, lifted my spirit up, literally put a smile on my face.

Through Grace I received much love, friendship, caring and

support from her friends in Rossmoor. I attended countless parties, participated in bible studies, church activities, Chi gong club, Ballet club, Ping pong club, Line dancing club, the Chinese American Association of Rossmoor, Chinese Performing Arts Association. With CPAC support and the sincere and professional guidance of my Peking opera teacher Jacie Wang and lovers of Peking Opera in the Bay areas, I reestablished a Peking Opera Club in Rossmoor. We successfully performed three shows for the community. My valuable Peking opera teacher, Bao Qi-long, still enthusiastically coaches me on line every week. The love and uplifting energy from all these activities are the blooming flowers giving the inspiration and beauty to this community. I was like a booming flower, respected and loved by people. Indeed, Grace is the most beautiful flower in my life's garden. Her kindness, generosity and friendship helped me to get beyond the mental trauma in an unbelievably short time.

Grace helped me to get back my laughter and smiling face. How can I not to feel gratitude and thanks to the universal Devine whose energy wave lead me, uplifting and willing, to do more for this world!

When Daniel was going through his hard time, Dr. Liu Li walked with me every day when I was in the most pain. She accompanied me and encouraged desperate Daniel. His five sisters came to visit us every week by turns, especially Sara and Annamaria, who even came to stay with me until their brother passed away. In order not to disturb our friends and invite more sorrow for myself, I chose not to tell people about Daniel's advanced cancer situation. However, Jane Shaw, Nancy Zhu, Tom Wang, An Li, Xiao-yan Zhou, Yuan-feng Zhang and Katie Wang were all able to visit us one week before Daniel left this world. I will be forever grateful to these friends, but at the same time I felt guilty to other friends for depriving their chance to say good-bye to Daniel, whom they have held in high esteem.

My relatives in China over 30 were sad for Daniel's leaving but are now less worried about me.

Living in this beautiful garden of Rossmoor, I am like the bud of a flower blooming healthily and beautifully. Apart from my old friends in my life, I have also made quite a few new friends. I am happy every day. Not only because there are more than 200 clubs and my hobbies can find a home here, such as table tennis, tennis, ballet classes, Qi gong classes, golf courses, wonderful indoor and outdoor swimming facilities, a concert hall, cinema theatre, all kinds of ball room dance parties etc., Yet the most important are the people around me. They are like a beautiful strand of pearls. Or to mix metaphors, each one of them is like a flower in full bloom in the garden of my new life. Because everyone who lives here is in their retirement years. There is no competition or struggle. To live happily and healthily are the only goals in their life. Everyone is upbeat, active, sincere and friendly. I always feel I am already in my paradise, surrounded daily by enchanting music and poetry. My way of thinking has reached another level. I realize that the love I had experienced and felt in the past was so limited. There is no comparison with what I have felt and experienced now. I understand more about love, friendship, the relationships between people. It seems I have gained a completely new world view. Friendship and love are the most valuable qualities of human beings. It doesn't allow pollution, dishonesty, or misunderstanding. It doesn't allow expectations or selfishness. Any doubts or selfishness will injure or ruin the most valuable qualities of human beings. There is none of that here.

We are not relatives but are closer than relatives in many ways. Sincerity, kindness, and selfless dedication are my mottoes now. My friends are my soul mates. They are my spiritual food for thought.

Among all my friends, not only have I encountered multi talented people, such as Anna Veneziano, an accomplished lyric Italian soprano from Italy who is willing to teach me western singing technique; Maggie Chan a very accomplished pianist from Shanghai, China who enthusiastically accompanies me when I need her, I also have received guidance and enlightened instruction from the psychic masters who have opened their third eyes, such as Reverend Charlotte Tinker and Qi Gong Master Antonio Morrocco.

Somewhere, sometime, they miraculously came into my life. I can talk to them about anything in my mind, and they are able to point out the road in front of my feet and guide me so I won't go astray. I am really blessed. Even though I have stepped towards octogenarian age, I am still full of infinite yearning and beautiful longing. I firmly believe I will complete my life circle in this paradise-Rossmoor which is only 20 to 30 minutes-drive to my daughter's home. Her home has her husband, my son-like son-in-law, my two lovely and multi-talented grandchildren. It is my harbor, the source of my happiness and my full support in every aspect of my life. I always feel I am the luckiest lady in this world.

Chapter 20

Grateful

"Grateful for every little bit of water-it nourishes me

Grateful for every flower that brings me fragrance

Grateful for every white cloud which weaves my dreams

Grateful for every ray of sunshine which holds up my hope

Grateful to my parents for giving me life

Grateful to my teachers for teaching me to grow

Grateful to the people who helped me appreciate their kindness

Grateful to those who hurt me which let me learn to be strong

Living in a world of gratitude, a world of harmony and beauty

Living in a world of gratitude, a world with you and me"

When I heard the two lines of the lyrics, "Grateful to the people who helped me to appreciate the kindness, and Grateful to those who hurt me which let me learn to be strong," I was amazed by the events that had happened to me recently. I changed my plan to learn Western songs from Ms. Zhou, my voice teacher. I told her that I wanted to learn this song :"Grateful." The lyrics were written by Mage Zhengxing, music composed by Mr. Wang Shengli, sung by Zhong

Liyan, a student from Guan Mucun, a famous and accomplished alto singer in China. It was recommended to me by my friend Y.Y.

The more I studied this song, the more I realized the profound meaning of Mage Zhengxing's incisive words. The more I sang this song, the more I felt the beauty of Mr. Wang Shengli's melody. Teacher Zhou's teaching, inspiration and guidance enchanted me and I can't stop practicing singing it several times every day.

Since my husband Daniel passed away, I have had the privilege of meeting many people who are kind, sincere, and helpful since I moved from Pebble Beach to Rossmoor at the invitation of Grace Wang.

Here I would like to write a few touching stories happened to me recently. I want my readers to share with me the sincere feelings, warmth and friendship of this world. It also serves as the closing chapter of the English version of my autobiography.

First of all, I would like to talk about Li Ning and Zhang Peiyu. They are husband and wife. My three girlfriends and I booked plane and boat tickets for a trip to the Danube River in Europe. When I checked in at the San Francisco airport, I realized that I did not bring my own passport, but Daniel's! The plane would depart at 2:30 and check-in would close at 1:30. It was 12:30 p.m. then. I immediately called my friend, Zhang Jian, who took us to the airport. I asked him to come back to the airport and take me back to Rossmoor where I live to get my passport. However, it would take at least 80 minutes to make a round trip. We had to cross the Bay Bridge back and forth! I was about to miss the flight! I suddenly thought of my mentor and Chi gong teacher Antonio who will help me to bring my passport to the airport. But he was receiving acupuncture treatment in Oakland.

He came up with an idea: to find a friend in Rossmoor who knew my home and could rush to the airport with my passport. I thought of the kind and enthusiastic my Beijing folks, Li Ning and his wife. As soon as they received my call, they rushed to my house to get my passport, and quickly arrived at the airport.

The American Chinese manager at the airport also took special care of me. I checked in at 1:50. When I appeared at the boarding gate, my three girlfriends who were anxious and worried about me were overjoyed. Thanks to the help of these friends, we were able to embark on our unforgettable riverboat trip to the Danube in Europe.

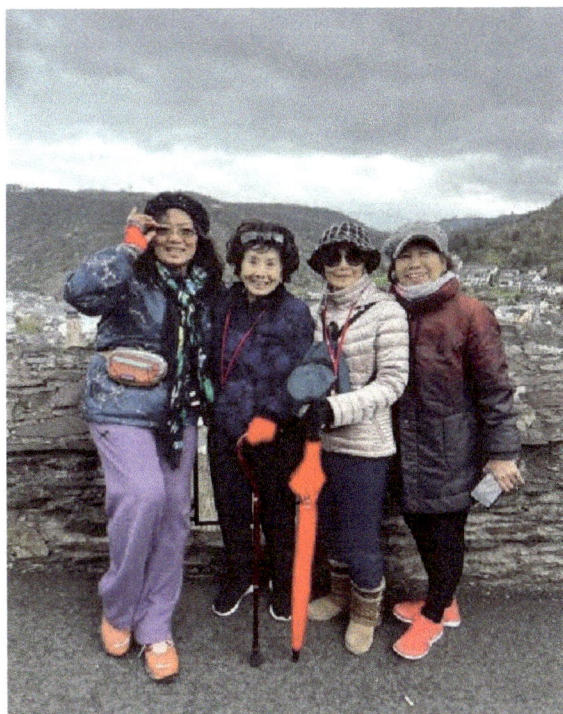

My travel girlfriends Mei, Grace, Jane and I

Secondly, on May 18, with the full support of the Rossmoor Chinese Performing Art Club, the Rossmore Peking Opera Art Salon in which I am the leader successfully performed a traditional Chinese Peking Opera repertoire for more than two hours.

Among the nearly 30 performers, I invited several professional orchestra payers and professional Peking opera singers in San Francisco Bay Area to join the show. After more than two months of rehearsals and everyone's efforts, we overcame all kinds of difficulties and presented more than two hours of traditional Peking opera programs including "Happy Dragon and Phoenix", "Zhao's Orphan", "A Precious Bag of Jewelries" "Mu Guiying in Command", and "The Palace of Eternal Life", as well as the orchestra's ensemble "Spring Festival". The audience highly rated our performances.

During the rehearsal, I was very moved by Ms. Von Deman, who played The emperor of Tang dynasty. Although she is not a professional Peking opera singer, she has studied and performed all her life. In Taiwan, she is honorably known as "Meng Xiaodong." (a famous Peking opera female singer who played the part of a male). This time, she warmly accepted my invitation and "accompanied" me to play the part of Emperor Tang Minghuang in "The Palace of Eternal Life." I was deeply touched by her dedication to art and her diligent study of every word and every line. In order to make the performance a success, she stayed at my house for three days. Every day we rehearsed the lyrics until 12 o'clock at midnight. I am very grateful to her.

She also asked me to go to Taiwan in December this year to perform. I am looking forward to it.

Here are some good reviews for our performance.

Richard Schulman, who had studied Chinese and Tang and Song poetry at Yale University and later taught at Harvard University was extremely excited after watching the

performance. The next day he took out the Chinese materials he had studied to review Chinese, and also found Bai Juyi's "Song of Everlasting Regret". Mr. Schuman also asked his wife to tell me that he understood the whole story. (We only played a scene in the whole play). His wife, Lydia, (the same first name as mine) played

one of the four chamber maids in "The Palace of Eternal Life" in which I played the Royal Concubine). Lydia Schulman is the only American in the whole performances and I owed many thanks to her willingness to play a chamber maid despite the language barrier. She also acted as the stage manager in the last minute to help the smooth communication behind scenes.

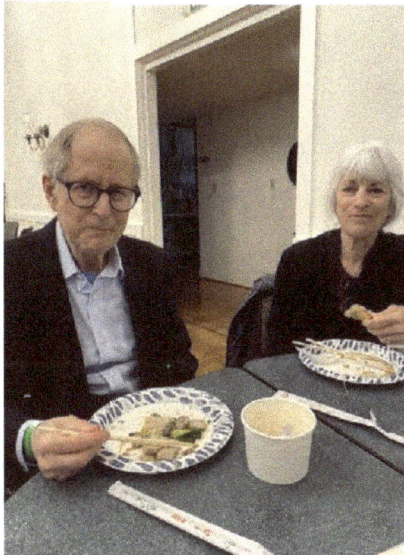

Richard and Lydia Schulman

Another Chinese-American expert on Kunqu Opera and Peking Opera, Li Linde, who was a professor teaching Kunqu at U.C. Berkeley and also translated the famous Kunqu play "The Peony Pavilion" into English came to watch our program with her brothers and sisters from all over the world and gave us full recognition. We thank her for coming and proud of ourselves to get approval from an expert.

My mentor and Chi gong teacher, Antonio Morrocco who used to visit the Metropolitan Opera House in New York frequently when he was young said, "I never thought that you could organize such a successful Chinese Peking Opera performance in this place in California. From the professionalism of each performance, the use of lighting, the slide captions of both in Chinese and in English , the fabulous color of the costumes, the makeup, the coordination of the staff and the effect of the orchestra, I feel as excited as entering the Metropolitan Opera House in New York. "

On the second day of the show, I met an 88-year-old dentist in the gymnasium who was also a marathon runner. She grabbed my hand and said, "I didn't expect your performance yesterday that successful. I took my neighbor to see your show.

She excitedly told me that she had never seen such a wonderful show in her life. It was indeed beautiful. You should consider doing it again next year. "

I am very grateful to God to give me this opportunity, and to the teachers who have taught me Peking Opera for many years: e.g. Dong Xiayu, Jacie Wang, Qian Qiming, Bao Qilong, Lu Juan. I am also grateful to the orchestra and all the people in my group for their support and encouragement.

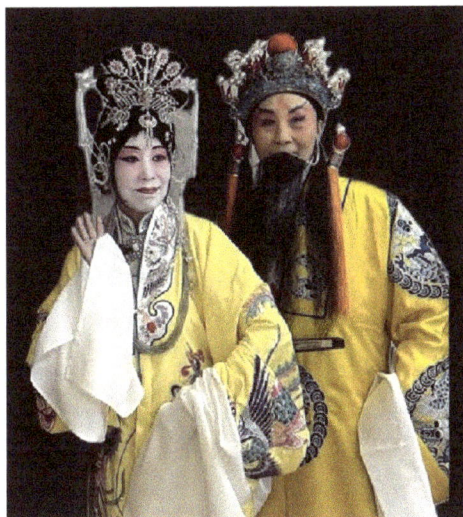

With Von Deman

She played the Emperor I played the Royal Concubine

The third story is: on June 24, I had an operation because of a malignant carcinoma on my right thenar. My friend Cao Yanfang accompanied me to the hospital. Thanks for such a good friend!

When I was chosen by Bai Xuemei to perform with her the 24-style Tai Chi Umbrella at the Tai Chi Club on July 9, I was diagnosed of the malignant carcinoma on my right hand.. As soon as she heard that I was going to have surgery, she said we should cancel our performance. But I didn't want to fail the expectations of Xu Yansheng, the director of the club, so I persuaded Bai Xuemei to let me continue to practice with her. Xuemei came to my house every day to cook for me and clean up the kitchen. I was very grateful and also made a request: I was afraid to look at my wound and asked her to help me change my dressing every day. She did. In addition, Y.Y. and others also helped me change my dressing. After a three-day break, Xuemei and I continued to learn the 24-style Tai Chi Umbrella. We successfully completed the performance task on July 9th and ived up to the director's expectations. Actually, I could have followed Xuemei's advice: cancel the performance. But I thought of a famous saying in China: What matter most, for the Buddha, it is to receive an offering of a stick of incense; What matter most to a person, it is he/she should live to its fullest as long as he/she has one breath. I never quit! Under Bai Xuemei's great efforts and careful care and to pick me up and back forth to practice the form almost every day, the two of us successfully completed the performance task. I'm going to sing aloud, "Grateful to those who helped me appreciate their kindness." Thank you Bai Xuemei!

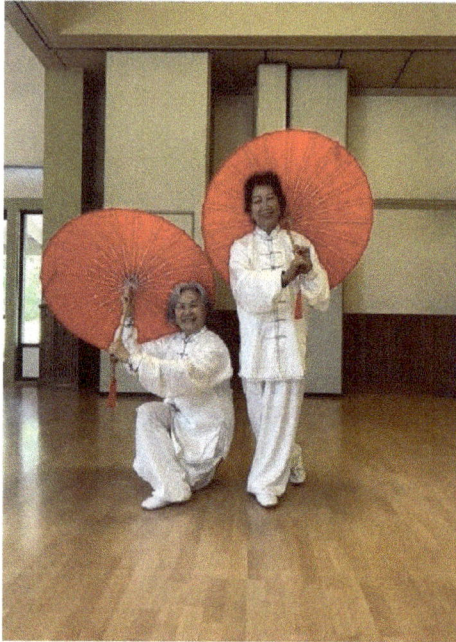

With
Baixuemei

The last story is even more unbelievable.

On July 22, Monday I went downtown to meet a friend but I lost my purse. Inside there are all my ID, bank cards, health insurance cards, and dollars. When I got home, I sat on the couch and don't know whether to laugh or cry. I was blaming myself for being careless when the phone rang. It was from the police. After the officer checked my name, I couldn't believe my ears when he said, "Your lost purse with Audrey Hepburn's picture was brought to our police station. Are you going to pick it up or you prefer we send it to you? " I asked, "Really?" Who sent it?

Where did you find it? " I was overjoyed when the police officer (who also went by the last name Li) handed me my purse, which I had lost for five hours. I checked it, and there was nothing missing. "You are truly God's favorite". This is true of what a good friend once told me.

On the third day, I met this lady who sent my lost purse to the local police station. Her name is Itzel Martinez. She works in a men's high-end clothing chain store downtown Walnut Creek.

She told me the story when we met: At three o'clock that afternoon, she went out to take her lunch break and saw a beautiful purse on a bench on the side of the road. There is an avatar of Audrey Hepburn on both sides of the purse. At first she thought someone had dumped an old purse. She picked it up and took a look. "When I opened it, Wow! There are all kinds of cards for one to live in the United States. There were also dollars inside the small purse. I waited for about 5 minutes and wondered why the owner had thrown such an important purse on a bench on the side of the road in the downtown area. Nobody showed up. So I decided to send the purse to the police station after my work." I said, usually people would take the money and throw away everything else. She said that my education and my heart did not allow me to do that. 'Tm wondering how anxious the owner would be. Now I'm glad the wallet is back in your hands." I asked her if her manager knew about it but she didn't tell anyone. I approached the manager of the store and told him the story of his employee, Itzel Martinez and how grateful I was.

They should be proud to have such an honest and kind employee.

Through the loss of my purse event, I owe many thanks to the two bank managers of Wells Fargo and Chase. I rushed to their offices right before the closing time and told them the story and request them to cancel the ATM cards. Aaron Lee Medema of Wells Fargo and Amany Mahrous of Chase Bank not helped me right away regardless the office hour but also called me the next day to check with me what else they could do even though they were told I had my purse back.

There are many very disappointing things happening in this world. Some people said the morality of human had dropped to the lowest point in history. However, from what I have experienced so far I have to say the majority of people are still kind and with high standards for themselves.

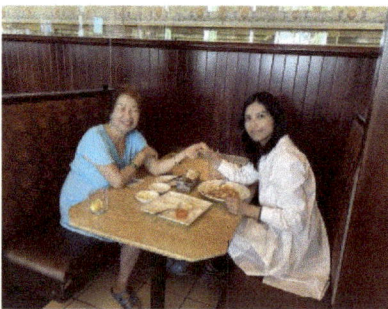

With Itzel Martinez

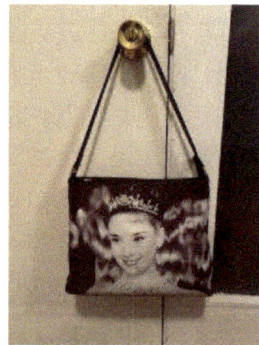

my lost purse came back

Now I'm going to sing aloud, "Living in a world of gratitude

This world of gratitude is harmonious and beautiful

Living in a world of gratitude

This world there are you and me."

people.

People used to say, "The sunset is beautiful ,

but it is just near dusk".

However, I would say, The sunset is beautiful,

I am not afraid of near dusk.

I am grateful at my old age I have met so many nice

May good people be blessed

Life is like a marathon, as long as we persevere, we will eventually reach the other shore in our hearts

Annex one

Testimonials from Readers for the Chinese Version

When I first started writing this family history and autobiography, the purpose was simple: to let my friends and family members understand how I spent my life. In my old age. It is also very gratifying to recall the road I have traveled. Our descendants of the Li family have no idea what their ancestors were like. Writing it out also gives them a little bit of understanding of their ancestral origins. After the first draft, I showed it to my relatives, classmates and close friends. They gave me many pertinent suggestions to make the whole article more in-depth. I didn't expect that I received full affirmation and praise. Several of my friends in the United States told me that they cried while reading my stories, and they had drawn many inspirations. I think this "autobiography" has no longer my personal experiences. I decided to publish it. With their consents, I have selected the feedbacks and attach them as an Annex to share with you, my dear readers.

"After reading the autobiography of the Third Girl, I was very moved. Three words, true, kind, and courageous. True: Authentic life, not mixed with the false emptiness of the vanity. Kindness: See your kind heart, tolerance, patience, always praise others, not a sign of ordinary Chinese who are often envious and jealousy. Courage: After so many tribulations, your bravery and unyielding spirit eventually lead to positive results. As a Manchu woman, I especially understand your temperament. Nothing can knock you down. You have been crawling and gritting teeth to get through the difficulties. Thank you for your painstaking efforts to revise the work. I'm proud of you. Way to go!"

- Wang Shu-mian Former Assistant Professor of Defense Language Institute USA, Xiang Hui

I carefully read your autobiography and felt very deeply moved! Thank you very much for being open and bold in showing us your true self completely and unreservedly! I like your personality which is cheerful, kind, sincere to people, helpful for others, have a strong desire to learn, a wide range of interests and hobbies. You can sing and dance, do not meet the status quo, pursue higher ideals, a lifetime of learning new knowledge! What touched me the most was the process of your tenacious struggle against the disease, the spirit of fighting with it to the death, overcoming the unbearable pain and suffering beyond ordinary people can endure and finally enjoying life health, happiness and the joy of life! So happy for you! You described your three marriages in details, and we finally understood how much they loved you! Love the three men in your life ! People always think that everything is ready for you when you come to America, which is a fantasy! Your American experiences are the history of life struggles and ups and downs.

Your happiness has come. Bless you! Love and take care of yourself. Thank you!

- Chen Su-cun Former Senior Lecturer Xi An Foreign Trade School

"I have finished reading it. Very good! Your autobiography is written smoothly because I know you too well. I feel it is very real, and a vigorous, bold, and hard-working Li Xiang-hui (Li Chong-jun) is presented to us.

- Zhang Gui-Zan Former Director Foreign affairs Office He
Nan University

"I have completed the reading of your memoirs. It is indeed a masterpiece. Thank you for allowing me to get a better understanding of your personal life. It is a lucky thing to make you a worth trusting friend. It is my sincere wish that you will enjoy the rest of your life as happy as you used to be."

- Wei Zi-bin Former Oklahoma Trade Representative

"Li Xiang-hui,

Your memoirs truly described the self-improvement, tenacious struggle, creation of happiness, cultivation of positive results, and your inspirational life displayed that the "Third Girl of the Li family" has gone through ups and downs for more than 70 years! Praise for the extraordinary life and fighting spirit of special stunts!"

- Zhang Yi-feng Former General Manager of Development
Department of CNIEC

"The change of dynasties of the Third Girl, the collision of tradition and new trends, changed your conservative personality, and created your desire to chase new things. You can plant seedlings early in the rice, and you can also be diligent in the autumn harvest, and hard work has forged your strength. You're handsome and delicate, but not shy. Playing all kinds of ball games, swimming, skating, gymnastics, you have done them all and shine yourself to the world. You are rebellious, abandoned the old world and left your family to join the tide of youth going abroad.

You are brave, the trauma of the Cultural Revolution did not let you sink and resolutely broke into the Western magic garden. The pressures of the family, the gossip of society, the torment of the disease all seem to have nothing to do with you. The optimism of nature allows you to go through the clouds and see the sunrise and enjoy the unique happiness of your old age. You are "debauched" bohemian , unwilling to be lonely, uneasy with the status quo, going your own way, and have to be an unusual self.You stop at the remnants of the Manchu Qing Dynasty, walk on the road of a fantasy western world. You have won life, and you have won countless eyes to look up. I sincerely wish you good health and well-being in the days to come! I am very happy to read the masterpiece. From time to time, the memories are still fresh in my mid. Excuse me of my helpless pen clumsiness and beg for forgiveness.

- Chen Zhen-yu Former General Manager China Resources

"Hello Xianghui! I finished reading your autobiography. It was so touching! Very vivid and beautifully written! You have the courage to liberate yourself, have a great personality, pursue your ideals and happiness, and do not seek perfection without grievances. There are not many people with character like you! Very accomplished! This life of yours has not been in vain. You are outstanding among our schoolmates. I am very touched after reading it. I believe that other students will have the same feeling if they have the chance to read it!

Am I allowed to send it to other students to appreciate? Thanks again for your autobiography!"

- Xu Wei-qiang, Schoolmate

"Autobiographical essays revealed the myriad states of China's political system and interpersonal relationships with her own experiences. The Tang Dynasty monk and three disciples went to the Western Heavens to get the scriptures of Buddhism. All the way they went through great hardships, descended demons and caught hydrocarbons to obtain the True Scriptures. It seems that you also have three companions to bless you to go to the Western Heavens to take the True Sutra and become a Buddha. When you are alone you handle yourself well and when you are accomplished, you are kind to the world. May the Buddha bless you and everything goes well."

- Richard Zh Former Director of Tian Jin Free Trade Zone

Vice General Manager China Petro Wuzhou Petro Import

export Co. LTD.

"Your Manchu family lineage part describes the encounter and real life of the ordinary People of the Manchu people after the emperor was expelled from the palace, which is very touching. I saw the picture of flag emblem of Manchu Eight Banners for the first time, and the character, life ethics, and family relations of the Manchu you described are very insightful. You are a woman who pursues Chinese cultural knowledge unremittingly, have a high cultural accomplishment, involved dance, Peking Opera, martial arts, music and other aspects, and become a messenger of Chinese culture in the United States in the colleges where you teach and the communities where you live, and are respected and loved by people."

- Zhang Yulian (Zhang Xian) Former Director of Translation
and Editorial Division
Director of Meetings and Publishing Division of the United
Nations

"Reading your revised masterpiece gave me a lot of thinking. I can't imagine that you had spent so much effort and time into this writing. The work is quite rich in contents and very sincere in feelings. Later, many precious photos of historical significance were added, making the work fresh and real, and then more or less reflecting the color of the times. The work is in the form of a memoir, which unabashedly expounds the pain and happiness on the road of your life for decades."

- Wang Yinsen Schoolmate

"Today I am particularly sleepy and at six o'clock I went back home for dinner but did not want to eat. I wanted to go to sleep right away, but before going to bed I habitually browsed WeChat and saw your autobiography. When I read about your optimism and strength during chemotherapy and your love story with Gene and Daniel, I was moved to tears several times. I want to express my feelings: Daniel regards you as the most beautiful woman in the world! Even when your hair is thinning during chemotherapy. Even when you really don't have hair like a nun, I see you as beautiful as ever! That kind of beauty emanates from the depths of the heart, insightful, confident, strong, loving, open-minded, simple, kind... I don't know what other words can be used to describe you. You say, "Life is a big stage. Each of us is an actor on stage. Whether you play the main role or the supporting role, whether you play a tragedy or a comedy, the audience will cry with you, and some will laugh with you. Some may appreciate you, some may not want to see you, and some may not care at all. When you're done acting, the play is over, and your life is over. " I would like to say that life is like a drama, and a drama is like life. I remember that a few years ago, after you read my writing you encourage to write my story. Now I suddenly have the urge. You are the most wonderful woman I have ever seen in real life! The love between Daniel and you is a true love that is purer and more touching than the love stories in novels and movies! How many men in this world fall in love with a woman when she has cancer recurrence and chemotherapy, and doesn't have a single hair??? It is a love without any impurities! Thanks for sharing!"

- Kiki, Friend

"Your friend seems to be a talented lady with stories, and like you, she is also a literary person. She is right, you are a beautiful, strong and atmospheric woman, and what touched me most about you was that you could still face your students and friends without hair that women love the most."

- Yu Zhen-gang Friend

"Dear Lydia,

Only after examination can life be meaningful, and only then can we know more clearly whether the pain of the past can be faced and can be understood so as to let us calm, relieved, let go and accept. Your autobiography reflects a lot of Chinese and American history, culture, as well as different realms of ingrained traditional Chinese thoughts as well as the free and open Western lifestyles. Yourself are a perfect combination of Chinese and Americans. You pursue high in the spiritual world, self-disciplined, and self-cultivated. Your face is full of stories, but there is left no wrinkles or worries. You are always full of vitality and you are a woman with the best state. As your close friend, I am proud of you, but also admire your eternal persistence in pursuit of art. On the journey of one's life, you are brave and tenacious, dare to say and dare to act. Your heart is clear and transparent. You came to this world for your ideas. To love needs courage, to give up, not only needs greater courage, but also needs to be confident. If one only kisses the shadow, he can only receive the illusion of happiness. On the road to love, you not only became to know yourself, but also found yourself and the result is beauty belongs to you."

- Guo Mei-sheng Assistant Professor Defense Language Institute
USA

"Today I finally finish reading your masterpiece! There is only one sentence to express my feelings towards your ideas and writing: "Admire to the extreme." Although you have experienced some great tribulations in your life, you are brave and resolute in face of difficult situations. Thus the flowers blossom and bear good fruit after storms. Congratulations!"

- Jane Shaw Dormer Professor of Defense Language Institute
USA

"Thank you for giving me this autobiography as special birthday gift. I have finished reading it and benefited a lot! The life of my third auntie is magnificent. Your struggle and success manifested the value of your life. You are indeed my idol!

I wish you : Eternal like the moon; Boundless energy like the rising sun; longevity as of the mountain and pine trees, it does not collapse; Good luck and happiness are with you!"

- Ye Chun Nephew

"It's a great autobiography and family history, enriched with a lot of content, pictures. The writing is wonderful and smooth, like a novella. Thank you aunt!

- Tian Wen-shu, Nephew, Senior Arts &Crafts Artist

"Very powerful my talented and beautiful third aunt. Seeing your tenacious struggle against the disease during your illness, I know how difficult it is for you. Everyone's patience is limited, but your patience is admired by everyone - and all your desire to learn is also something we must follow. We all should take you as an example, learn endlessly, live to learn and the most important thing is that your mentality is very healthy and high. I'm proud to have an aunt like you."

- Ma -Xiao-hua, Niece, Office Clerk

"Dear sister, your autobiography has been written for several years and finally came to an end. Allow me to borrow some sayings to express my feelings towards you: the old roots are strong; the scorching sun leave the leaves even greener and the old horse is ambitious for thousands of miles. In the long years, I have also encountered many bumpy and tortuous roads and suffered a lot of grievances. Although life is not as rich as you, I am still like a small grass, under the nourishment of the sun. I have experienced the spring, summer, autumn and winter in my life. However, this is the character of our Manchu women: tenacious and gifted. We are enthusiastic and cheerful, kind and virtuous. How affectionate is the term of "sisters", which contains blood and kinship! You are the coffee and I am the cup. You are the leaves and I am the branches. Mom is the root of this big tree. The feeling of our sisterhood is growing deeper and deeper by each day. My blessing to you comes true from the bottom of my heart. They are just like thousands of rivers and mountains that last forever and my care for you is forever. I wish you are in a good mood every day! Wish your good fortune like the east sea and your longevity is like the pine tree!"

- Li Chongxiang, Sister, Chief Accountant

"After reading Li Xianghui's masterpiece "The Bitterness and Happiness of the Third Girl of the Li Family" in one breath, I was really touched! When I recalled the editing of "Don't Forget the Road to Come" in 2021, I was shocked by the stylish and delicate writing of Professor Zhang Yin-yu by Li Xiang-hui my school sister. In particular, it is written vividly that Professor Zhang issued an inner soul cry in the depths of the red wood forest, which is the final release of a generation of intellectuals who have been precipitated for too long! In "The Bitterness and Happiness of the Third Girl of the Li Family", the same shock comes from the author's inner true exposure to three marriages and the extraordinary mental perseverance of treating cancer twice. As the author frankly admits, a person will encounter a lot of people who love you or the opposite sex whom you love. One has to follow the call of her heart, but at the same time always be grateful to the lovers in her life. Unfortunately you have to endure the infinite grief caused by separation. If the content is categorized separately, such as family, education, three marriages, cancer, etc., as well as more details on farms and factories life , this masterpiece will be read even better. I sincerely wish school Sister Xianghui good health and much happiness!"

- Hao Bao-sheng, Editor-in-chief International Trade Forum

"Brother Hao: I am happy to read the praise and approval from the chief editor for Li's writing. Li Chong-Jun's story is touching. Compared with most of the old five years' schoolmates in Beijing Foreign Trade institute, her experience is not the most complicated, but the ups and downs she experienced have their own characteristics, which have a lot to do with her emigration to other countries. In particular, the huge impact of family love and physical health on the depths of a weak woman's soul is heart-wrenching. This person's innate tenacity makes her not bow her head, not to yield, her teeth are crushed and swallowed. Her life has been very full of stages, and reading her words makes you anxious for her and makes people sincerely admire."

- Ho Lin-sang Former Manager China Headquarters
Standard Chartered Bank HK/Singapore

"Among the old five year students of Beijing Foreign Trade Institute, there are many ups and downs in the second half of their lives. Your memoir makes people sigh thousands of times. The girl in a Manchu family, ten fingers had never touched anything in the kitchen and was spoiled and raised like a baby. In old Beijing, it is commonly known that nobody dares to bother the ladies in Manchu families. Although you have not cultivated a domineering character, the strength of not bending and not willing to admit defeat is vividly reflected in your life. I like a sentence by Mr. Lu Xun: First, people must survive, and second, they must develop. Your dedication to survival and development is impressive, whether it is in any land, or for personal careers, or love and family."

- Ho Lin Sang Manager China Headquarters
Standard Chartered Bank HK/Singapore

Annex Two

Quotes from Readers Who Read Chapter 20

"The emotion of gratitude writing is sincere and touching, which fully demonstrates your attitude of gratitude in the face of adversity. Each story is full of human warmth, conveying kindness and mutual help between people. You use simple language to describe the kind people you meet in your life, and give back to these good things with a grateful attitude. The article not only makes people see your strength in life's challenges, but also inspires us to cherish every help and care around us, be grateful, and convey warmth. After reading it, my heart was also filled with gratitude for life and admiration for the beautiful humanity. " (from Meisheng Guo)

"You are such a brave, lucky and happy person. I am happy, saddened, and proud of your situation. Your life is full of passions, joys, ups and downs, and tribulations, but you never give up hope, and you are always so strong to face everything and pass it peacefully. Wishing you a peaceful, healthy and good life for the rest of your life. " (from Jane Shaw)

"Your perception is very transparent! You enjoy writing and see the brilliance of humanity! The words shared by those who have reached this state will definitely help and influence more people. " (from Zhongqing Zhang)

Photos:

A complete gallery, mostly in color is presented at:

www.LydiaOlson.online

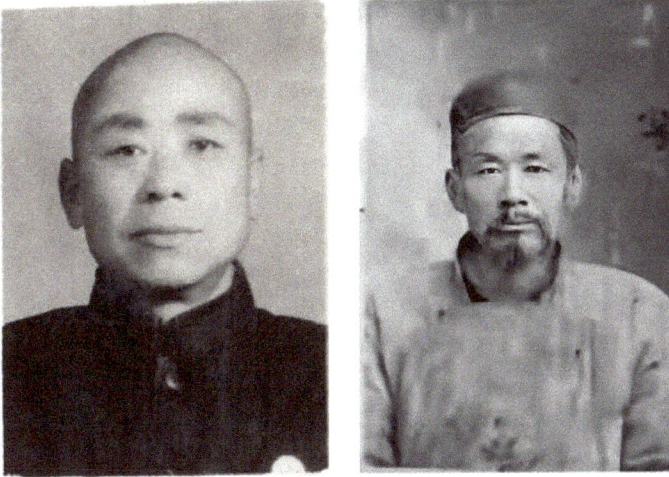

My Father (left) and Grandfather (right)

My Family (of Manchu origin) on next page

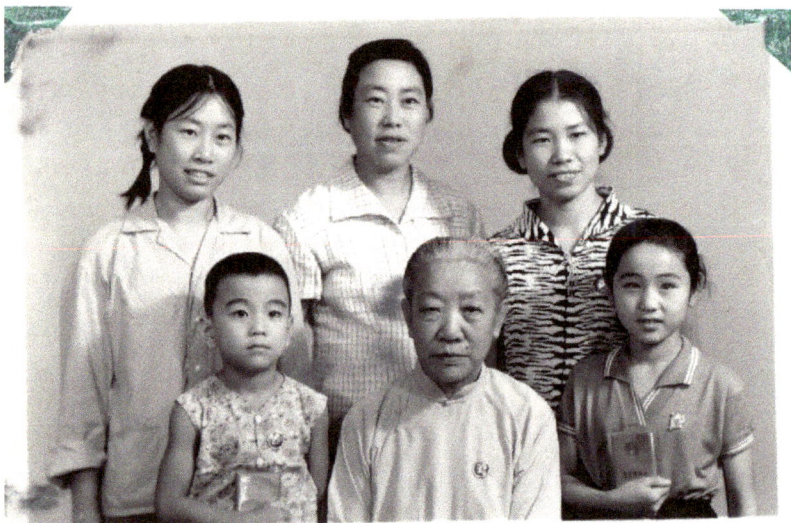

Mother and children... I am at top right.

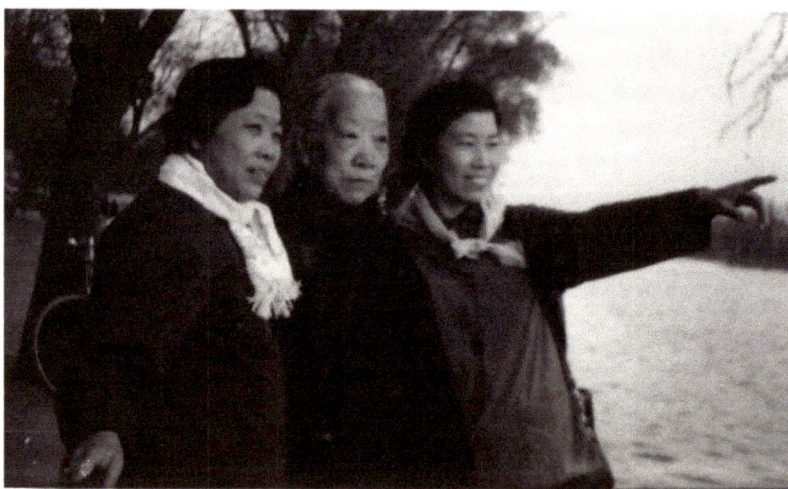

With my Mother (center) and Elder Sister (right)

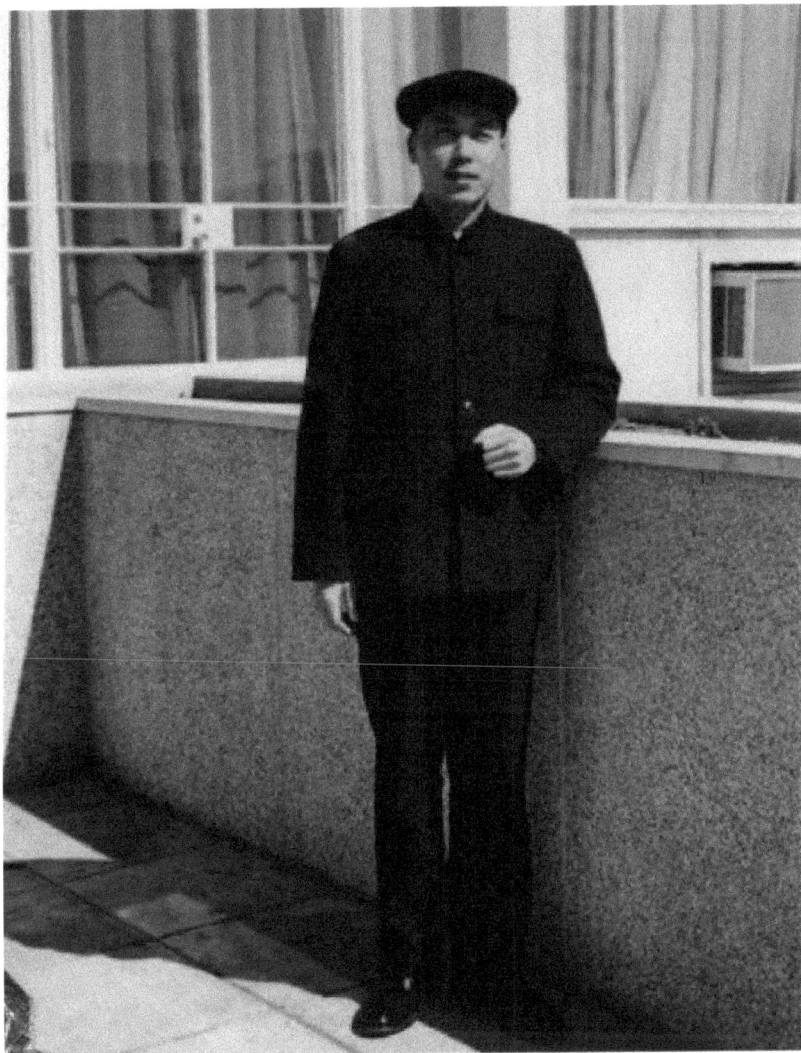

Bingshen, my first love and husband.

See all the photos!

More Photos:

A complete gallery, mostly in color is presented at:

www.LydiaOlson.online

9 798986 684598